Losing Aaron

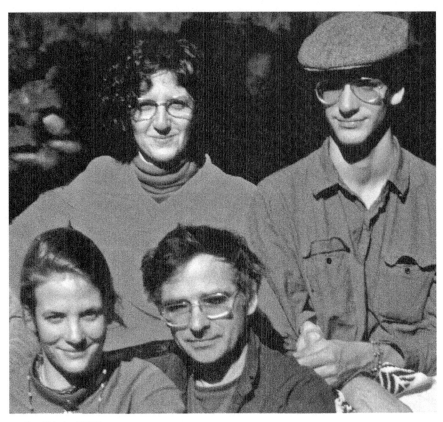

In Ojai, 1987
Back row: Ingrid and Aaron
Front row: Stasha and Arthur

Losing Aaron

A Memoir

INGRID BLAUFARB HUGHES

Irene Weinberger Books

Copyright 2016 by Ingrid Blaufarb Hughes
Irene Weinberger Books, an imprint of Hamilton Stone Editions,
    P.O. Box 43, Maplewood, New Jersey 07040
ISBN 9780990376736

Names: Hughes, Ingrid Blaufarb, 1945- author.
Title: Losing Aaron : a memoir / by Ingrid Blaufarb Hughes.
Description: Hamilton Stone editions. | Maplewood, New Jersey : Irene
    Weinberger Books, an Imprint of Hamilton Stone Editions, [2016] |
Includes
    bibliographical references and index.
Identifiers: LCCN 2016006004 | ISBN 9780990376736 (alk. paper)
Subjects: LCSH: Schizophrenics--Biography. | Schizophrenics--Family
    relationships--Biography. | Mother and child--Biography.
Classification: LCC RC514 .H84 2016 | DDC 616.89/80092 [B] --dc23
LC record available at https://lccn.loc.gov/2016006004

Book design by Susan Hood
www.SusanHoodDesign.com

Chapter 1

My daughter took the call. It was a Saturday in April of 1999, and I was just getting out of the shower, looking forward to a quiet day and then a quiet week with no classes or student papers to read. As I was reaching for my clothes, I heard footsteps pelting down the stairs. Stasha was crying, yelling.

"Mom, Mom, Mom."

Why is she so histrionic? I thought, striding through the bedroom to throw open the door.

"A woman from the embassy in Paris called. They found Aaron's body hanging from a tree."

Stasha is so irritating, I thought, and at the same time, No, it can't be, we'll talk to him and explain he doesn't have to do this. I tried to picture Aaron in a tree. But I couldn't.

Taking up the telephone to call Paris, I was half-aware of a familiar tension in my spine, a burden of fear and anxiety. Stasha and I sat on the bed as I punched out the long number she had written down.

"American Embassy."

"This is Ingrid Hughes. Someone called me about my son."

"One moment, please. I'll patch you through."

Holding the phone to one ear, I sat on the edge of the bed, my arm around Stasha, crying a little, staring at the brick hearth of the defunct fireplace a few feet away. The bricks had black scorch marks from long ago, but they were scraped naked now, the fireplace barren and empty.

The duty officer came on. "Mrs. Hughes?"

"Yes."

"Your daughter told you?"

"Yes."

"The police found your son hanging from a big tree in a park about noon." Now I could see it. The big tree. Aaron's long, narrow body hanging.

"His body is at the city morgue."

"At the morgue," I repeated stupidly.

"I'm sorry it took so long to let you know," she said. So long? It was still Saturday morning, I thought, forgetting the time difference.

"If you want to get him back, you'll have to wait a few days to get hold of an undertaker. Easter Monday is a holiday here, nothing will be open till Tuesday." What does she mean, get him back? Isn't he dead? I wondered vaguely.

"Are you sure it was Aaron?" I asked.

"The police were sure. He had his passport with him. They wanted to know if he was depressed."

"He had a mental illness," I said. "What's the name of the park where they found him?"

"Parc des Buttes-Chaumont." Automatically, I wrote down the unfamiliar words to look up later.

2

"I'm so sorry," she said. "I'm so very sorry."

Stasha and I sat on the bed for another moment in the quiet of the large white room, its tall windows looking out on the skeletal ailanthus trees. Two days earlier Aaron had been with us. Active and functioning in his own way: tall, handsome, hostile, competent, articulate, nasty at times, convinced he was being poisoned and lied to, but in the last few days calmer. I held on to my sense of his warm body, his living, breathing presence. It would fade, I thought. But for now I had it. He had been here. He had been with us.

Then he had set off for Paris in a blaze of fury, making what I thought was another of his many round-trips across the ocean or across the continent since his illness struck.

Now he had hanged himself. Even years later those words shake me. He was gone. Gone irrevocably. Gone by his own choice. He lay in the Paris morgue—a body, no longer a person.

Yet I had seen daily the pain he lived with, the disappointment, his continual anger, bitterness, anguish, the effects of an illness that had battered us all. I knew why he had taken his life.

My first understanding that Aaron had lost his mind came in the spring of 1992, seven years earlier. I was living then in Brooklyn, in the studio I had taken when I left Arthur—left him despite love and respect, despite our long history together, going back to our time at boarding school in Colorado. Our youthful marriage had been the ground we grew up on; our familial foursome had been the greatest satisfaction of my life. But Stasha and Aaron were grown now. My love for Arthur felt like one of those rivers of the canyon lands, a river that had worn away rock over the ages and flowed in a narrow channel through layers of ancient history. The passion that carried me away from Arthur was a spring flood, a deluge of water and snow melt, dislocating ruthlessly anything in its path.

A flood does not provide an easy transition. I often felt insecurely rooted in my new life, though my plan was clear. Days I was tutoring at the Reading and Writing Lab of Baruch College, my first job since college. Evenings I was pursuing a degree in teaching English as a second language at Hunter College. A better job lay ahead when I had my master's.

Aaron was in his first year of a doctoral program at MIT. Physics had been his pleasure, his preference since high school. He enjoyed it and excelled at it with an ease that was characteristic. In high school and college, he had been remarkable for his striking competence, his even keel, his humor and good sense. But on a recent visit, he had dissolved into tears, crying inconsolably as he sat across from me at the tiny table where I had served our breakfast. The trigger for his outburst was a mention of an embarrassing episode in his first year at Swarthmore, four years earlier. But his misery was so great I thought there must be more to it.

He agreed to see a family therapist with me, Ellen Wachtel, the person Arthur and I had talked with during our last months together. Stasha and Aaron had met her too.

"Ingrid and Arthur didn't prepare me for what I want to do," Aaron told Ellen. Though Stasha called us Mom and Dad, Aaron had always called us by our first names.

"They were never successful." This hurt. How could it not? It also puzzled me. His education had been excellent, first at private schools where he had the freedom to study math and science in his own omnivorous way, and then at one of New York's special high schools for science. He had graduated with distinction from Swarthmore and been accepted by every doc-

4

toral program he applied to. With his friends and his teachers, he assumed the same attitude of respectful equality as he did with us. Yet now he felt we hadn't provided what he needed. Though I could see his distress, I couldn't make sense of it.

Later, I saw Ellen again on my own. She made it clear she considered Aaron shaky. "Help him hold himself together," she said.

On the phone one Sunday evening early in April, he seemed particularly disturbed and discouraged.

"You sound upset," I said.

"I am upset."

"I'd like to help."

"You want to help," he said dubiously.

"Yes, I do."

But he didn't see how I could. We said good-bye.

Despite his obvious unhappiness, despite his recent outburst of tears, despite Ellen's assessment, I was unprepared for what came next. A few minutes later, he called me back.

"Maybe you do want to help," he said. "And maybe you know that when I walk on the street people are making fun of me—in an organized and systematic way."

Fear shot through me. With that one sentence I knew he had crossed the line into madness—into a world of his imaginings, a world far from ours. What was real to him was plainly impossible to me.

"Aaron, it seems that way to you. These perceptions aren't accurate. That's not happening," I said. "We'll get help." I don't remember what else I said, just the electric fear in my body, the pressure along my spine.

I called Arthur and was glad he was at home in the apartment on East 9th Street. His companion, Lanie, was an old friend, but I didn't want to call him at her place right now. I repeated Aaron's words to him. He was upset, of course. But he left it to me what to do next. That had been the pattern of our marriage, and especially of the decisions we made as parents.

In the morning I called Ellen Wachtel. She gave me the name of a psychiatrist in Boston and encouraged me to go to Aaron for a few days.

"What if he won't let me? He's been so distant and angry."

"Tell him firmly you're coming," she said. Her support helped. I needed to be with him. When I told him I was coming, he made no objection.

During the days till I could leave for Boston, I walked around in an odd state of shocked languor, as if I'd been gutted and lost my core. My spectacular son had been struck by mental illness—my generous, confident, brilliantly able son.

At work I coasted along on empty. The other tutors were talking about some news they found disturbing.

"I just expected more," a young Trinidadian woman said as we sat together during our break.

"Uh-huh," I said. Finally I realized that the verdict had come down in the Rodney King case; the ensuing outbreak in Los Angeles was part of the background of the next few days, a headline in a paper on a newsstand, a radio report I caught in passing, or a scrap of conversation.

Tuesday evening I had a visit from Jay, who was the reason I had left Arthur. As I told him about Aaron, his brown eyes were serious, his large forehead furrowed. Meeting his gaze, I was conscious of my fear and a sense of inadequacy in the face of

Aaron's illness. Through the lens of my anxiety, I saw Jay too as lacking. He knew how proud I was of Aaron. He had a sense of him from me. But he had met Aaron only once, very much in passing. How could he understand what I was feeling?

"So you're leaving Thursday morning?"

"Yes. I'll be back Sunday."

"I'll give you Jan's number. Maybe you can stay with her." Jay had friends in Boston, where he had lived until our relationship pulled him to New York.

Before I left, I called Stasha at her apartment in Brooklyn. "I'm going to Boston. Aaron has had a breakdown," I told her. At twenty-six, she was two years older than Aaron, but it wasn't her job to deal with his illness—it was mine and Arthur's.

As my train pulled into Boston's South Station, I reminded myself of Ellen Wachtel's advice to be matter-of-fact, not to probe or make it harder for Aaron by acting upset. I stepped onto the platform, my daypack on my back. Aaron stood at the front of the train, tall and straight in a tweed jacket and dark jeans. He turned away, rather than watch me approach him, rather than meet my gaze. I reached up to embrace him, and he gave me a wisp of a hug. His jaw bulged because he was clenching it, changing the shape of his face, and he was so thin the muscles of his shoulders and neck had shrunk.

From the station, we walked to Boston Common along sunny streets crowded with lunchtime strollers.

"I've been to this place," he said, and leaned against the wall of a restaurant, while I gradually realized he was suggesting we eat there. As we sat at the table, his features were often contorted, angry, uncomfortable, even crafty-looking. When he wasn't grimacing, tension lines on his face made him look older than his twenty-four years. He had been remarkable for his relaxed poise. It was entirely erased now.

The visible signs of his illness disturbed me, and I was glad he didn't bring up his delusions. They scared me, and I had no idea what to say about them.

"I got the name of a psychiatrist who's supposed to be very good," I told him.

"Arthur gave me a name too. Do you think it matters which one I call?"

"I'm sure they're both good."

After lunch, we wandered around the Common, watching the people in paddleboats on the pond, and sat on a bench under the newly leafed trees.

"How is your teaching?" I asked. His fellowship required him to teach a lab section.

"It's OK. The students are very worried about their grades. They're always bringing their quizzes to me to complain when I take points off for mistakes."

"Really?"

"They say, 'but it's just a little mistake.'"

"What do you say?"

"I just took off a few points."

When a child ran over and asked Aaron to return a ball that had rolled under our bench, he reached down for it and handed it over without a friendly word. This although he had always liked small children and been good with them.

Next morning, after a night at Jay's friend's house in Cambridge, I was happy to pass a deli where I could get good bread and curried chicken salad to bring Aaron in his apartment on Beacon Hill. It was sweet to have time with him. He let me lay my hand on his warm head, now and then, or his thin back.

"What are you thinking? You look sad," he said. This was the Aaron I had been missing, the dear, caring son I had brought up.

Riding back to New York on the train, I felt better. Being with Aaron for two days had restored some of my strength. Talking with him and touching him meant so much after the months when he had kept us at a distance, telling us not to call, barely responding to our questions on the rare occasions when he was willing to talk. He had agreed to see a psychiatrist, so I was a little optimistic. Yet I knew the crisis was far from over. His words on the phone—"making fun of me systematically and in an organized way"—were etched into me. His bulging jaw, his contorted face, his loss of flesh and muscle, all indicated he was seriously ill. But maybe not permanently. I had little knowledge of mental illness, but I knew some young people recovered.

Chapter 2

As I remember it, Aaron was ten or eleven when he became recognizably himself, the person we missed during the years of his illness, the Aaron we knew and loved. We lived then, in the late seventies, in Manhattan's quiet West Village, a neighborhood of brownstones and small apartment buildings lining streets that predated Manhattan's grid. Our apartment was on a five-sided block near the corner of West 4th and West 12th Streets: the first two floors of a small brownstone, a downstairs and an upstairs and a patio out the back door, like a little house, handily near the small progressive school the children attended on West 15th Street.

Aaron's first solo cooking project, when he was around ten, was making blintzes. Working from a cookbook, he taught himself to make the delicate pancakes he rolled around a filling of pot cheese. He cooked without help, standing at the stove, his blue eyes behind his gold-framed aviator glasses focused calmly on the skillet, his thick, fair hair a shining helmet. He turned the blintzes out on our plates as we sat at the table.

"This is good, but it isn't hot," said Arthur. With his broad forehead, deep-set eyes, strong nose, and narrow chin, he was a handsome man.

"Neither is mine," said Stasha.

"Nobody's perfect," Aaron said agreeably, and returned the blintzes to the frying pan for a few minutes. The confidence he brought to what he did was striking to me, the more so because it contrasted strongly with my own doubts and uncertainties. Even his relaxed, methodical cooking style was unlike my often-impatient way as I tried to throw a meal together too quickly. Unfazed by Arthur and Stasha's complaints, he still felt good about his cooking.

I have a note Aaron wrote around then:

I HATE TO NAG
BUT WILL YOU PLEASE
GET OFF THE PHONE
FIRST OF ALL I NEED TO
MAKE A CALL AND SECOND
OF ALL I HAVE TO GO SOON
AND NEED YOUR HELP!
   DON'T FORGET THE NEEDY

I saved it because it was clever, reusing the *New York Times* plea to readers at Christmastime, "Remember the Needy." There was also Aaron's tact—I hate to nag—and most important, his confidence that I would help him, if I knew he needed me. I didn't take his assumption for granted—it wasn't a feeling I had enjoyed growing up.

My own parents, I felt as a child, had little sense I needed them and less ability to help as they carried me around the world, from London to New York, from Greece to Bethesda, Maryland, from there to Saigon and then Singapore, where my father worked at the American Embassies. During those years, I was crowded from my domain as first by Nora, David, and then Billy, feeling increasingly that I barely merited my parents' attention. Often, when we were abroad, their time was taken up with Embassy social life, its welcoming parties and farewell

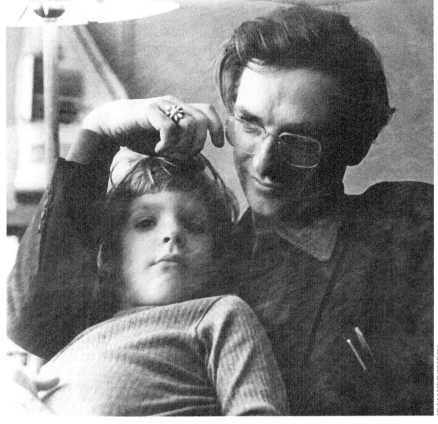

Aaron and Arthur, 1975

parties and no-reason-at-all parties. My parents seemed to me to slip ever farther off, like twin planets whose strange orbit carried them only away, never closer.

If my father was home after work, he would take off the jacket of his linen suit, loosen his tie, and sit reading through his thick glasses. He never talked about the events of his day, nor asked about ours. My mother was busy with my younger siblings or with volunteer work. Reading enabled her to shut us all out. "I just turn off my hearing aid," she would say happily, describing her ability to block out our voices when she had a book in her hand. Growing up, I thought she was different from my friends' mothers because she was English: her old-fashioned bun and severe sheath dresses, her remoteness, her suspicion that strong feelings were self-dramatizing made me see her as the mother of few words, the one who didn't explain, who came from an earlier time and an older place.

When Stasha was born, my most conscious goal was to be utterly unlike my own parents. They had been distant; I would be there to talk about whatever my children brought up. My parents had lived a silence that stifled understanding. Lacking a vocabulary for my emotions, I grew up bewildered by them. I would tell them who I was. I would listen to them and know who they were. Through the years my sense of being different from my own parents never left me.

At twelve, Stasha would go off to Friends Seminary one day, looking stunning in my new dress of red flowers on a black ground, and the next in her own snug jeans. She looked very much like Aaron. Her blond hair was short then, and like Aaron she wore glasses.

I knew a day or two before her first period that it was coming, by the way she described what she thought was a stomachache. The next evening she called me to her in the bathroom.

"Mo-om." I found her sitting on the toilet looking suspiciously and without pleasure at the stained crotch of her underpants.

"Is that my period?" she asked accusingly. I assured her it was, then ran downstairs for a package of pads. Arthur was just coming in from work.

"Stasha got her period," I said. When I had provided her with clean underwear and one of the pads, I gave her a big hug. She looked at me in gloomy amazement.

"Congratulations, Stasha," Arthur said quietly from the door. I was glad he had acknowledged her period, making it something that could be mentioned.

"I don't see why everybody's so excited," she said.

"Are we going to the bank?" Arthur had promised Stasha he would take her to open a savings account during the bank's late hours. ("Getting her period is like having money in the bank," our friend Lanie Fleischer said on hearing the story.)

For a couple of days, Stasha was all cool avoidance. When her façade broke, she flung herself sobbing onto my lap.

"Everything's awful." Tears streamed down her cheeks. "I hate our house. I hate school. I hate my teachers."

"But you got such good reports," I said.

"I don't care. I hate them anyway. My friends are terrible. And I *hate* having my period." I rocked her in my arms, relieved that I could hold her.

When she had cried herself out, she relaxed and dried her eyes. "I wonder if tears are good for your complexion," she said.

"Stasha is lovely and wonderful," I wrote, "but she has to struggle so much more than Aaron." She was my first, my daughter, born when I was just twenty. I saw myself in her, not always my best self, but my conflicted and uncertain self. I was hard on her. "Stasha sings doo-wop continually and swivels her hips and practices her dance steps in front of every available mirror," I wrote with irritation rather than amusement.

About Aaron I wrote to a friend: "Maybe Aaron will be one of the new men. He is so smart, so helpful, perfectly beautiful with his big bones and symmetrical body, and all that blond straight hair, always looking inside things, seeing how they work, telling me how, looking at maps so he knows where we are on the earth."

Arthur, in parallel fashion, had more trouble with Aaron. Stasha asked me one day, "What was the name of the Greek king who kills his father? That's what Daddy and Aaron remind me of," a remark we laughed at for many years. Despite this Oedipal friction, Arthur and Aaron were good friends. They worked together to set up Aaron's electric train track, fastening it to a piece of plywood hinged to the base of Aaron's bedroom wall, so it could be folded out of the way.

With my children I was the person I wanted to be: loving, connected, sharing my days with them. I felt Stasha and Aaron almost as parts of each other, the two people I had given myself to most fully, whose lives I had shaped, and who shaped me in turn.

In the beginning I was so proud of their baby bodies grown within me, then fed by my milk. "Look at Stasha's legs," my mother said admiringly when Stasha was a toddler. "They're like little trees." First Stasha and then Aaron rode on my hip, or lolled on my lap, climbed on me, hung on me. As they got older, I often snuggled with them at bedtime. When Aaron was

15

nearly as tall as I, he would stand behind me, so I could bend over and lift his weight draped down my back. When I could no longer lift my children, they would pick me up. "Stand still," one of them would say, and hugging me hard, raise me a few inches from the floor.

I knew that when my children's intelligence and good temper switched to sulks or anger, it didn't take away from their essential goodness. I trusted them to love me and accept me. This was not how I felt about myself. My sense of my own failings was continually undermining, despite my therapist's reassurances. How I relied on my therapist; how I loved her for leading me out of the desert of my self-hatred.

I was working on a book about the daily lives of parents and their children, an idea that had seized me when I saw that my ideas of how children should behave had more to do with my illusions about Other People's families than with the realities of ours. But Other People had many of the same difficulties I did, I realized at a school parents' meeting. I decided I must shed light on my new discovery: reality! What I had grasped, the world must need to learn; with the grandiosity of the utter novice, I saw myself writing a Studs Terkel–type book of interviews on family life, revealing the daily ordinariness of parents' lives with their children.

Let me resist the urge to mock myself. My subject was a good one. It was one of the important issues opened by that time of reexamination of women's lives. Having children had been the first choice of my adult life and remained central. But that didn't help me put together the book I envisioned. My interviews with mothers and fathers went well, I thought. But it was much harder to shape my material. How had Studs Terkel done it? I fumbled and hesitated and finally reconsidered, deciding fiction based loosely on the families of the people I had interviewed would work better.

With Arthur I often felt insecure, in part because of my own history, in part because his commitment to the Socialist Workers Party felt like the heart of his life. At SWP headquarters, he was working on the party's lawsuit against the federal government for spying and harassment, a suit which succeeded in exposing details of the FBI counterintelligence program of surveillance and disruption of groups on the left.

Arthur had been born into the bourgeois society he often reviled, as the great-grandson of John Murray Forbes, whose wealth had come from the nineteenth-century shipping industry, and especially the China trade, which forced opium from Turkey on the Chinese in exchange for tea to sell in the US. Arthur lived uneasily with the conflict between his political convictions and the inheritance that allowed us to live so comfortably. When we vacationed on the Forbes family's Naushon Island, a short boat ride from Woods Hole, Massachusetts, he sometimes felt uneasy with his cousins.

Aaron and Stasha enjoyed our times there. Once I helped Aaron as he measured and sifted flour for a cake. As he beat the batter, he sang quietly to himself, "You Light Up My Life." When the cake was ready, I set it on a tray with glasses of milk for the children and a full pot of tea for me and Arthur. With a whelming up of happiness, a sense of abundance, I carried it to the table. What good fortune we had in having each other, in being together in this beautiful place.

"It would be nice to be friends with my cousins," Arthur said as we drove back to New York. "But when I talk about what I really think, they aren't interested." Occasionally one was even a bit shocked to discover that there was a socialist in the family.

In New York Arthur kept his wealth as inconspicuous as he could when he was with his political friends, referring vaguely to Naushon as "the Cape," if he mentioned it at all. His contribution of a substantial chunk of his inheritance to the SWP was known only to a few.

Like Arthur, I felt the corruption of our society. But at times I felt he used the SWP as a shield against my needs or the children's. I resented his long days working at party headquarters, since I saw them as voluntary, while Arthur considered them to be a requirement of his work. At better times I knew he loved me and was grateful for his steady acceptance of my ups and downs, his warm hand on my skin in the dark, holding me to him.

Much to my dismay, in 1979, when the SWP was urging its members to take industrial jobs, Arthur got work at Metuchen Ford in New Jersey on the Pinto assembly line—on the night shift, no less. By the third day, I dreaded finding Arthur rousing himself in the darkened bedroom in midafternoon, his eyes red, as he pulled himself out of sleep to prepare for another grueling night at Metuchen.

Aaron too found the thought of Arthur on the assembly line upsetting. Now and then through the evenings, he would mention him. "I bet Arthur is saying, 'Oh no, here comes another Pinto.'"

I felt for Arthur as well, though I didn't see how it could be necessary for someone with his abilities to stand riveting a piece to the chassis of a car over and over all night long. How could a person as reticent as he become the spark that would ignite change? I'm sure I misunderstood the role he saw for himself, I was so disturbed by what he was doing. I knew there were people who worked on the line all their lives. But they had to. Arthur didn't.

We were all relieved when Arthur quit after a few days. In the fall he took a job as a pipe fitter at the Brooklyn Navy Yard, assigned to work on the USS *Seattle* in dry dock. By then I was resigned to his taking a job in industry. Working during the day was more realistic. He would often be home for supper and the evening. The Navy Yard was also easier to get to, just over the East River in Brooklyn. I could live with this.

Chapter 3

Aaron was in fifth grade, getting ready to change schools the spring that Arthur worked briefly on the Pinto assembly line. I prepared for his transition by putting together a list of progressive schools in Manhattan and Brooklyn Heights. Once we had visited three or four, he knew where he wanted to go.

"I like Calhoun," he said. "I like the way the teachers and students talk to each other." At eleven Aaron already had an authority about him that inclined us to accept his choice.

"You'll have to take the subway," I said.

"I can do that."

When I got up in the mornings, I might find Aaron sitting at the table working on a model sailboat, a project of his and Arthur's, or loading his books into his pack. As I got breakfast, he often made his own lunch. Stasha would rush in, eat a bowl of cereal, and dash for the 14th Street bus, which would carry her across town to Friends Seminary. Aaron and I would sit talking till he collected his watch, his dimes, his pack. "I hope I catch an express train at 14th Street and it passes the local," he might say, describing the subway commuter's ideal ride. And off he would go.

At Calhoun Aaron met Philip Lidov, another bright, blue-eyed, fair-haired youngster with bangs, and they became fast friends, visiting back and forth after school. Philip said later that Aaron's presence in sixth grade had rescued him from the "typical eleven-year-old boys who had not yet found much to interest them other than sports and the testing of each other's vulnerabilities. Aaron had already found many more things in

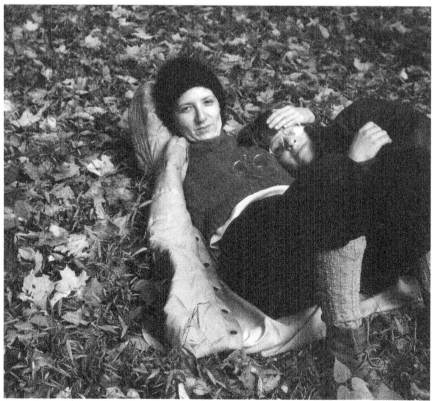

ARTHUR HUGHES

Ingrid and Aaron, 1978

which to be interested." Aaron treated all those interests—his math and science, his electric trains, his books of optical illusions, his collection of Agatha Christie mysteries, his school projects—with the same focused, relaxed intelligence.

In a letter to a camp friend I found in his notebook, Aaron described the trial of the shah of Iran held by the fifth and sixth grades.

> I was the prosecuting lawyer. I've been researching for the past month, getting eye-witness acounts and facts for the trial. There were 2 charges, the first, robberry, and the second, torture and murder illegally. We had 5 sets of jurys, all had unnanimous votes of guilty for murder and torture. 3 said guilty and two were hung jurys for robbery. All together the whole thing was a lot of fun.

Aaron must have heard us talk about the Iranian revolution. But he did his research at Calhoun without consulting us, as a project he shared with his teachers and classmates. I was aware of it only when his teacher, Sam, mentioned it during a conference. I drank in Sam's praise of Aaron thirstily.

It happened that Philip's father had the next conference. Sam introduced us by our names, not our children's.

"I'm Aaron's mother," I told him, like an Arab woman introducing myself as Umm Aaron, my feminist principles momentarily blown away.

This was a time when I was working in my therapy on recognition of my own strengths and pleasures, and solidifying my comfort with my own happiness. But I remained uneasy if I praised myself, perhaps in my writing group, uneasy if I was too happy, too pleased with myself, and liable to tip over into anxiety. But being proud of my children, praising their abilities and accomplishments gave me no trouble at all.

Stasha picked up Aaron's math book and tried to demonstrate that it wasn't really a seventh-grade book, introducing many of the concepts she was studying in eighth grade. But when she was assigned an essay about a family member, she began, "My brother is good at science and math. My brother is good at everything." Then she laid down her pen, stuck.

"I can't think of anything else to say," she told me. Finally she switched to my mother as her subject and wrote a charming and insightful portrait. But it was hard having her younger brother shine so while she fretted about essays or tests. She was a good student, smart and hardworking, yet often anxious and doubting her own ability, and then cranky as a result. Still she had a deep generosity and a fund of good sense.

In 1980 Arthur and I bought 311 East 9th Street, a beautiful old brick house built for one family more than a century earlier. We occupied the first floor and the basement, slightly below street level. Tenants lived in small apartments on the top three floors. While Arthur would have preferred not to be a landlord, he agreed that paying an exorbitant rent made no sense. For me our names together on the deed made another connection, providing a security I hadn't known I wanted.

Our upstairs rooms had high ceilings, tall windows, and grand marble fireplaces. The living room even had afternoon sun. In the garden, two ailanthus trees had managed to grow as tall as the building.

"You certainly live like members of the ruling class," said one of Arthur's fellow SWPers, a young woman given to just the kind of hyperbole Arthur had feared. He didn't seem upset, but I was irritated.

With his friend Andrew, Aaron would visit the stores that sold early home computers, where they could play with them as much as they liked. Keeping up with developments, he saved up and bought himself a Commodore 64. Our television was his monitor; tape cassettes provided memory. Sitting usually in his bedroom, with its French windows opening onto the garden, he worked at the computer with complete composure. He never got upset and told the computer it was stupid if something didn't work. Instead he tried it again, and if it still didn't work he figured out why. When he produced something he particularly enjoyed, he would call anyone nearby to see it.

"Isn't that neat?" he would ask, sitting happily at his little table, as a graph of sine curves appeared on the television screen. To me, it was all magic.

The four of us sprawled on Arthur's and my bed as I retold the story of Aaron's birth for his fourteenth birthday. I did this every year, first for him in January, and then for Stasha in February, in celebration of their arrival in our family. Aaron's thick hair was cut straight across his forehead; there were traces of childhood plumpness still in his cheeks. His gold-rimmed glasses framed his eyes.

"I woke up early in the morning," I said, reciting the story that was familiar to all of us. "It was still dark. Arthur drove me to Beth Israel. We were in the middle a bitter cold spell, and it was very, very cold outside. At the hospital, the doctor started the contractions. They were intense. Arthur was right by me, wiping my forehead and giving me ice to suck. When I thought I couldn't handle the pain anymore, the doctor said, 'You're ready.' They wheeled me down the hall to the delivery room. Arthur and the doctor and the resident were all standing down at my feet. I pushed and I pushed. I remember I got a charley horse in my calf. And then you were out, and the doctor held you up by your feet and said, 'It's a boy.' And they let me hold you before they took you to the nursery.

"Next morning I could hear them rolling the baby bassinets along the hall, but they didn't bring you. So I got out of bed and asked for you. 'We wait for the new mothers to have a nurse to help them with their first feeding,' the nurse said.

"I know what you're going to say," Aaron said at this point. "I'll tell Stasha, just as proof." He whispered in her ear.

"I said, 'This is my second.'" He smiled and put his hands over his face. How sweet he was, I thought.

"So they brought you and I nursed you."

The day after his birthday, Aaron came home from school to find me in bed with menstrual cramps. I might have been reading a book I intended to review for a little paper in New Jersey, *New Directions for Women*. Or perhaps for *Motheroot*, another feminist periodical. Aaron sat himself on the floor near me and held up a purple plastic alligator, a wind-up toy from his friend Nicki at school. He opened it up and began taking it apart.

"What are you doing?" I asked.

"Open heart surgery."

"How's it going?" I asked a little later, looking up from my book.

"It's whole body surgery now," he reported cheerfully. He put it back together, wound it up, and let it chug along the floor.

———

In eighth grade, Philip applied to Stuyvesant High School, on East 15th Street, just a few blocks from our house. Aaron went with him to take the entrance exam.

"Do you want to go there?" I asked.

"I don't know." He paused. "It's so big. It has three thousand students. I don't know if I want to go to such a huge school."

"You can stay at Calhoun if you want."

"Yeah. But Philip is going. Joel is going too. Stuyvesant is a good science school."

Aaron fell into silence, his expression uncertain. He had enjoyed the atmosphere at the small schools he attended, and the freedom to move ahead at his own pace. But he chose to go to Stuyvesant, though he was sad on the evening of his last day at Calhoun.

That night he asked me to stay with him when he got into bed, a time when I would often lie down with him or Stasha to talk. Seeing his anxiety, I asked how his garden was growing—the imaginary garden in which he was supposed to grow good feelings.

"I'm growing broccoli," he joked.

"Where?"

"Here." He indicated his left shoulder.

I asked what he was growing in his pelvis.

"Moo shu pork. And lots of lettuce, an acre. And mustard and fortune cookies on my left hip bone." Then he seemed to feel better, and I kissed him good night.

Next morning I asked how his moo shu pork was growing.

"Very well." As we were getting breakfast in the kitchen, I caught him smiling down at me from his barefoot height, several inches greater than mine since just the past summer.

26

"Are you smiling because you're taller than me?" I asked.
"Yes."

Arthur seemed bored by his work as a pipe fitter at the Navy
Yard. The one bright spot was his pleasure in his coworkers. He
was happy when he cracked their deep Jamaican dialect and became good buddies with one or two. Sunday evening, as we sat
at supper, he would often sigh, look down at the table, and say
sadly, "Tomorrow I have to go to work."

I was glad when, in the spring of 1982, as Aaron finished at
Calhoun, Arthur accepted an assignment at the SWP headquarters on West Street overlooking the Hudson River. Beginning in August, he would be a copy editor at the *Militant*, "a
socialist newsweekly published in the interests of working people." We planned a family trip to Taos, New Mexico, where
Arthur and I had been married seventeen years earlier.

Our little vacation rental gave us a spectacular view of the
Taos Mountain, sacred to the Indians of the Taos Pueblo. Above
the mountain sailed a constant procession of towering cumulus
clouds, sometimes releasing rain in gray streaks that were
absorbed by the desert air before they reached the ground.
Occasionally rain would reach us, its pattering would turn to
pounding, and powerful cracks of lightning would strike. Aaron
took a wonderful night photograph of a lightning bolt one evening as we sat on our little porch watching a storm.

Malcolm Brown had been Arthur's and my art teacher at
boarding school, and a strong source of encouragement to Arthur, whose talent as an artist was apparent already in his teens.
Malcolm invited us for one of his vegetarian meals. When he
asked what we were doing with ourselves, and I explained that
I was writing a novel and also poetry.

"Ingrid had two poems published," Aaron said. I was happy that this modest accomplishment, which meant so much to me, had been significant to him too.

Across the red desert of Arizona and through the Navajo Nation, we camped at Navajo National Monument, which Arthur and I had visited as teenagers on a school trip and again on our wedding trip. Early in the morning, the four of us descended into the deep canyon, carrying food and water and overnight gear, our boots sliding in the sandy soil. In the ferocious dry heat, we hiked between walls of red rock along the trickling arroyo. Finally, covered with layers of dried sweat, we reached the ancient cliff dwelling, Keet Seel. A young ranger led us up a ladder to the cave whose tawny stone had protected the little village of adobe bricks built by the Anasazi people hundreds of years earlier.

Returning with our children to the stark, arid, beautiful landscape of Arthur's and my beginnings was a way of reclaiming the past. Back then I had been so terrified by my abrupt elevation into the status of wife and mother. Poor Arthur had borne the brunt of my frantic, crazed anxiety. I was always aware of my freedom from that anxiety, my satisfaction that I could now enjoy being with him. Being in this special place with Arthur, Stasha, and Aaron gave me joy.

"When you got married, you were pregnant with me," Stasha said as we celebrated our anniversary late in July.

"I was."

"Did you think about having an abortion?"

"Yes. But I'm glad I didn't, because if I had you wouldn't have been born. And I love you so much."

"Yes, I would. I would have been born later," Stasha said. It was comforting to know she felt there was no way she wouldn't have come to be the person she was now.

After our vacation Aaron flew west to hike the Cascades on the Pacific coast with friends. From Seattle he sent the seed of a birch tree, the tree of happiness, as the card accompanying it said. "You can plant this in your good feelings garden," he noted in a postscript. Stasha set out for the Wyoming Tetons. At home three weeks later, she reported what a good hiker she had been, keeping up with the strongest in the group. She wore her hiking boots around the city for days.

Home again I soaked in the city's energy. Musicians played blues outside the Astor Place subway stop. The library, the bakery, the butcher, the corner store, our Ukrainian coffee shop, Veselka, a clinic and a funeral parlor were all within a few blocks of our house. A subway token would get you to a museum or a concert. Everything you could need was here in the city—except the country.

We soon grew familiar with the rhythm of Arthur's weeks at the *Militant*: long days, with the longest on Wednesday, until nine in the evening, the night before the paper went to press, and the shortest on Thursday, when it was printed, and he got home at six. It was fun watching the paper roll off the clattering cylinders of the huge web press, which roared noisily and spit the collated, folded copies of the *Militant* out at the end of the line.

I dug into my current project, the story of a character named Greta Liebenbaum. Though I invented scenes and characters, the story of Greta Liebenbaum was the story of Ingrid Blaufarb. My taciturn mother and volatile father were hers. So was my adolescence in Saigon in the fifties, where I was indignant at my parents' absences and their replacement by four or five Vietnamese servants. At eighteen, as American troop levels in Southeast

Asia were escalating, I went for a job interview my father had set up for me. I presented myself to the secretary of the editor of *Congressional Quarterly*, who gave me a big smile.

"Ingrid Blaufarb. Your father is Doug Blaufarb at the CIA. I used to work in the mailroom there."

"If he is, I don't know it." I felt the ground shifting under my feet and sat down abruptly. My father, who had told us he was employed by the State Department, worked for the CIA. The father I had thought distant but candid had lied to me all my life, lied even recently, when I was old enough to know about his work. My conflict with him was a central issue of the novel and of my life.

There are writers who describe their parents' failings with humor, acceptance, and a degree of respect. How I would like to feel that generosity. Instead, for most of my life, I have thought of my father with a pained outrage. His belittling attacks on his children seemed to mirror on a familial level the American foreign interventions that he represented in his work—in Vietnam, in Laos, and as head of the Vietnam Desk at CIA headquarters. Granted, a sense of betrayal by our parents was common to my generation. Today, when young people more often want to get ahead in society than change it, it's hard to convey how energetically—and with what fury—we repudiated the world our parents had given us. For me the war—its toll of millions of Southeast Asians and tens of thousands of Americans, the lies that had created it and were its official face in the US; every fatherless child born to a Vietnamese woman and an American soldier, every shattered GI—engendered a lasting horror, some of which clung to my father for the rest of his life.

My novel was fed by my anger at my parents. At the same time, my writing deepened it. As I dismembered and remembered my adolescence, my parents' derelictions reverberated in my thoughts, fodder for endless therapy sessions and bitter tales I repeated to my friends. With indignant satisfaction, I seized on each new example of my mother's cluelessness or my father's demeaning attitudes. Yet I kept the subject of my novel secret from them, needing to protect myself and them as well. As I had since childhood, I maintained my own silence and told them little of what I felt about anything. Then I marveled that they didn't notice my reticence and held that against them too. Joking about them rather angrily, I called my father Captain Hook, my mother a sad, Victorian Mrs. Grimsby.

As far as I was concerned, my parents couldn't do right for doing wrong, to use a saying my mother produced when I complained that Stasha was being hard on me. My children provided the one unalloyed happiness in my relations with my parents. Often, when my mother was telling me stories about how smart or amusing my siblings' much younger children were, she would wind up by saying, "Keeping up the family standard," her way of complimenting me on my two.

Chapter 4

Aaron seemed nervous, starting out as a freshman among the thousands of students at Stuyvesant, but more aware of his uneasiness, I thought, and able to deal with it than when he was younger. In his last year of high school, he wrote a long entry in his journal about this time.

> The first day . . . I was happy but nervous. Philip and I were in the same homeroom. [The teacher] yelled at me . . . because I was talking. . . . I expected to be able to make friends and do well, and get along with my teachers. I was used to being happy and doing well at school.
>
> After the first marking period . . . I was petrified at the thought of not getting a 92 average, which my English teacher had told me was average at Stuy. And I didn't. I got something around 91.6.
>
> I got a terrible stomachache, the kind where its ok if you

are still, but it juts pain if you move. Immediately I started to think terrible things were wrong with me. Trichinosis? I became paranoid about eating pork that wasn't crisp all the way through. . . . I thought for a long time that on my hiking trip [that summer] I must have drunk some bad water. . . .

It wasn't all bad. There was still Philip and I enjoyed classes like Earth Science. I had high marks in science classes that I enjoyed.

As I remember it, Philip came over often, since our house was so near Stuyvesant, and the two of them soon had a group of friends. But at the time Aaron wrote this, he was trying to trace the development of his anxiety, especially about his health. Like Arthur, who had told me solemnly at seventeen that he had a heart condition, and also like Stasha, he was hypochondriacal.

On parent-teacher night Arthur and I divided Aaron's teachers between us. I walked up and down the halls, seeking out teachers in classrooms where the desks were fixed to the floors in rows in a school many times the size of any I had attended. The students impressed me as smart and energetic, living, I thought with some idealization, the life of the mind. Looking around Stuyvesant, I managed to forget that high school is about the social world as much as the mental. It's "a relief and a gift to have Aaron," I wrote, "who brings us ease and intelligence and success after success." A relief from my own self-doubt, I meant.

Arthur caught on to the Stuyvesant attitude better than I did. After overhearing other parents talking with teachers as he waited his turn, he said, "It was like watching a union negotiating session. 'Our daughter needs a ninety-five,' the parent says. 'She earned an eighty-nine,' the teacher says. 'How about a ninety-two?' the parent says."

The summer Aaron was fifteen, he and Philip and their friend Ben hiked a section of the Appalachian Trail. They plotted their route together, packing up parcels of food they mailed to post offices along their way. Philip's parents drove them up past Mount Mansfield in Vermont and nervously watched the three of them hike off along the Long Trail in their shorts and boots with their big packs heavily loaded. Philip said later that it was a hard trip. They were carrying too much weight, it rained a lot, their plan was too ambitious. Perhaps, like Philip's parents, we should have been worried that they were out of touch in rugged terrain. But we had a habit of accepting Aaron's estimate of his abilities. If he felt he could hike the Appalachian Trail with his friends, we thought so too. When Aaron called, he chatted cheerfully about their progress.

He wrote about the experience in his journal:

I had one of the best times hiking in Vermont. I felt at home and close to Philip and Ben, and free and happy. Excersize, good food, intimacy (with a few fights, but close fights). We tested our independence, we hitchhiked, we did a fourteen mile day. We impressed people. It was a blast. Going home was hard.

And in a school essay:

The emotions that come out of excercize are pure, unadulterated, and organic. When one is dealing with the material world, nothing lies.

The fall of his sophomore year, Aaron had many days when he stayed home sick, though often with nothing more than a cold or a stomachache.

Sophomore year I was miserable. My legs would twitch and wake me up, parts of my body would pulsate as I tried to go to sleep. Everything was wrong with me. The dots on my arms were lupus. Diabetes? Bio class did me in. Terror! Every syndrome I thought I had. My veins seemed really big—cholesterol build up? Tapeworm was a favorite—no wonder I was constipated. My arches were coming apart because of all the hiking—a degenerative joint disease! My penis hurt during orgasm—I had started masturbating early freshman year. Maybe something was wrong. I woke up in a cold sweat twice. Something wrong with my sweat glands. Maybe my intestine had a kink in it. . . . I got headaches—no blood flow to the brain. My sister was leaving [for college at the end of] that year, big fights. I had lost contact with Philip. Socially a wreck. Did I smell? Probably. For the first time I did badly in a class—bio. It terrified me. I was afraid of my body.

Reading this half-humorous conversation with himself, I am relieved to come to the final sentence: "Actually, I remember things at their worst." He did. But the depth of his fears, his nighttime sweats, seem significant.

As Stasha applied to college, I was her main support. Together we visited colleges for tours and interviews. I talked with her about her essays and went out for exactly the right shade of off-white Liquid Paper when she mistyped words on the application. Her first choice was Oberlin, where she applied for early admission. When the college deferred its decision till spring, she was weepy and dejected and in addition had to complete applications for other colleges. Head thrown back, her hand thrust into her thick, fair hair as if she might pull it out, she would storm in, announcing she couldn't do it! She couldn't do it— whether it was writing a paper for high school or finishing one of her college essays.

Perhaps one cause of Aaron's distress was her impending departure. At the age of three, at the time of Stasha's first sleepover at a friend's house, he had said, "I'm glad I don't have no sister. I wish I didn't have no sister all the time." And looked very sad when I put him to bed.

When he was eleven, he had been so pleased by the little birthday present Stasha got him I wanted to cry. He carried the yo-yo and the little jokes around the house, refusing to let them go even when he had to throw up.

Five years later he was so preoccupied by his real and imaginary ailments that by January I wondered if it might be a good idea for him to try therapy. I brought the idea up with him. But no, he did *not* want to see a therapist. He was sure.

And then, when he had a long weekend in January, he cleaned up his room for the first time in months and set up files for the schoolwork that had been lying in heaps on his floor. He approached his teachers to get into the most advanced honors math course and honors mechanical drawing. All so he could stay in the biology class he wanted. He spent more time working on his computer and wrote a program he submitted to *Compute!* magazine.

Though Aaron did well in all his science courses, his love was for physics and the math he needed to solve physics problems. "My interest in mechanical devices, and as a consequence mathematics and physics has become something I can always fall back on and always enjoy," he wrote. The long equations he left lying around the house were written half in Greek. He would readily provide an explanation we could grasp for what he was studying, so that his intelligence made us feel intelligent.

That spring he and his friend Peter came up with an idea for a solar-powered water heater, which they constructed in shop at Stuyvesant. It was a large sheet of metal bent in the shape of a parabola to reflect sunlight onto a pipe of water that ran at the parabola's focal point. Before they took it to Albany, they set it up on the street and then on the flagstones in the garden behind our house, where it stood for a couple of weeks, all six feet of it, its surface shining brightly under the ailanthus trees.

[A] friend and I entered a student energy research competition sponsored by NY State. We built a six foot parabolic solar collector and tested it out in the streets of New York City. Just having the chance and independence to design and build the complete project on our own was enjoyable. In the street, when we tested the collector, many people took an interest, stopping and talking with us. That was our first reward. . . . When we won second prize in the competition, it was satisfying to receive the recognition for the work we had done.

We all rejoiced when Stasha was accepted by Oberlin, since she had set her heart on going there. As the time for her to leave approached, I grew increasingly uneasy. She was so much part of my days. Would she want to be close to me once she was off on her own? As we sat quietly together in the living room, I wondered if she would feel that kindness to me was a burden, as I sometimes felt about my parents. I reminded myself that we were close friends, that she confided in me freely, that we had enjoyed many good times together. But I was always scared of being left, even when the person leaving was my daughter.

Together the four of us visited Iceland that summer, renting a car and camping out for ten days. We drove through the volcanic landscape, black sand traversed by streams of milky glacial melt, strange peaks and twists of basalt covered with the green, green mosses of this moist climate, under almost continual clouds. We swam in a hot spring and hiked through the miniature alpine birches.

At a little spot where we were the only campers, besieged by large angry flies, Arthur told Aaron, "Jump into the tent quickly so you don't let the flies in." Aaron pretended to be playing soccer with the flies, his long legs in his shorts moving quickly as he dodged and weaved. At Gullfoss, a vast waterfall, he got under my poncho with me to stay dry, though he now stood six inches taller than I did.

I had organized this trip because I thought it would be interesting, but especially because I thought Arthur would enjoy it. (Why? Why was it easier to think of a vacation Arthur would like than one I would enjoy?) Camping involved discomforts that I had a tendency to complain about. The ground seemed harder than it had two years ago in Arizona. Stasha accused me of being anxious. I thought she was too, she was so often impatient with me, teasing and even imitating me. Arthur remained his tolerant, patient self, driving us around, working with Aaron to set up our tent. Aaron made our breakfast oatmeal on our little camp stove.

In Reykjavik again, I found sleeping in a bed next to a bathroom with hot and cold running water perfectly delicious. But

Aaron had developed a headache that wouldn't go away and lay on his narrow bed, in the room he and Stasha were sharing, his head full of dire imaginings. Medical attention, we had learned, was the best antidote to his hypochondria. So a nice national health doctor came to the hotel and examined him.

"It's a headache," the doctor said.

"Just a headache?" I asked.

"Yes, a headache." He gave Aaron a mild painkiller.

"How do you feel?" I asked him a little later.

"Like I've been far away. But I'm coming back," he said.

From Iceland, Aaron flew on to Amsterdam for a bicycle trip through northern Europe. Stasha went to Mexico to study Spanish. When we were all home again, we viewed the slides of our trip. There we were—to my eyes all beautiful, and most beautiful together. We laughed at the image of me, caught by Aaron frowning ferociously from the front seat of the little car. But there were also pictures of us smiling happily.

"It makes you think we had a good time." Stasha said, and she and I laughed again.

"I'm never going to travel with you again," I told her without passion.

"Maybe when I'm grown up," she said.

Late in August Arthur and I drove Stasha to Oberlin, Ohio. In her dorm we helped her make her bed and begin her unpacking. Sitting on either side of her, we listened while the admissions director addressed the incoming freshmen. We rose when he asked parents to leave.

"I'm all alone," Stasha wailed, giving us a desperate look.

Hugging Stasha to me the next day, I had a familiar sense that I must have done something bad to deserve this loss.

———

At home Aaron volunteered to cook dinner for a week, making a different Mexican meal each night. He happily enrolled for physics, chemistry, and astronomy that semester, as well as English and Spanish.

He had bickered and competed with Stasha all his life. But when she was gone, he began a letter:

Dear Stasha . . . I haven't talked to you for so long, and I realize that you, someone I've lived with for 16 years aren't here anymore. . . . I think I've suffered, felt that your leaving leaves a gap. . . .

And then, when Stasha was back for midsemester break, he and she were friends in a different way. They went off together for lunch at Veselka, the Ukrainian coffee shop where we ate often. Aaron wrote in his journal: "Stasha and I have been treating each other like human beings."

My fears that Stasha would drift away were assuaged when I realized she wanted to tell me about her courses and her roommate and hear what we were doing in New York.

Junior year we saw a lot of Aaron's first girlfriend, Miranda, an agreeable youngster with a mop of curly dark hair. She and Aaron would chat with us or close themselves in Aaron's room. Aaron spent many afternoons working on an automatic gear-changer for a bicycle for another science contest. He spread his bicycle, his tools, and the parts he needed all over the battered old living room rug, staining it so badly I had to dump it later. But I couldn't bear to exile him to the cellar to work; I enjoyed

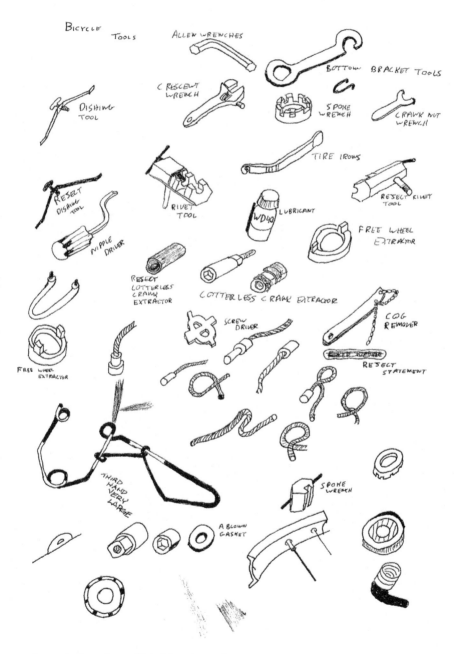

Aaron's drawing of his bicycle tools

his company so much. "My mother says she'll buy your gear-changer if you get it to work," Miranda told him. Aaron worked on it for long hours, but never got it going reliably. He submitted it to the contest anyway and won a prize. At the award ceremony in a midtown hotel, one of the judges told me, "We would have given it first prize, but we couldn't get it to work." Maybe that confidence to present your work, even if you know it's not 100 percent, is an important lesson.

After Aaron started Swarthmore, he told me that some of his physics teachers at Stuyvesant had suggested he compete in the Westinghouse Science Search, which offered a national prize for a science project submitted by a high school senior. But he hadn't wanted to, he said, long after the event. Why not? And why didn't he tell us at the time?

Chapter 5

In August we vacationed in Taos again. Aaron, preparing for his senior year at Stuyvesant, wrote in his journal while we were there.

8/17/85 I . . . think of Stuy and my conflict between doing really well like all the over-achievers and having more non-materialistic values. I'm trying to find a balance between my values and friends and my association between doing well and all the money crazed bastards who are going to Stuy to get an upper class job.

8/18 I pierced my ear today with Ingrid's not very helpful and Stasha's help. . . . I was surprised at how casual Stasha and Ingrid thought of it. Stash thought it was a good idea and helped pick the turquoise earing. I'll enjoy going to school with it—a new identity + self-assuredness—I think.

It was nice to talk with Ingrid about how she + Art were

when they were my age . . . Arthur feared success because of the bourgeoise values assosiation . . .

8/27 After I got my earing I had a fantasy that Philip would want to get one also, or would have one and it would be funny. Then I dread that he might think it stupid. I've got to have some faith in mys. . . .

8/28/85 I'm tense about my identity, my earing, how I'll respond to so desperately trying to be accepted. Now that I have some friends I think I'll . . . try to just be myself like I was this summer. Was I? Nervous about applying to college.

Here I am surprised by Aaron's suggestion that there was a time when he didn't have friends, by his desperate need "to be accepted." I remember that he often brought friends home from Stuyvesant.

Once school started again, he encouraged himself.

"I know I can handle all the work!!!! And the pressure!!!!!! He! He! He!"

9/1/85 Talk with Miranda and eventually she said she didn't want to be going out and I really could almost not speak. REJECTION!!!!!!!

9/2/85. Talked w/Ingrid and feel significantly better. I think I blamed myself almost completely for what Miranda decided . . . I hurt myself by not having a lot of confidence in myself and believing that I am a good person—which I am—a very good, understanding person who really knows a lot about relations and life.

9/10 Last night I slept well, really well, and talked with Ingrid this morning, and all was well. . . . Alls well that goes to the bathroom well.

9/12/85 Miranda and college have been two rather haunting issues for the past twenty-four hours. . . .

Aaron was happy when he and Philip went hiking over a long weekend. Yet his feelings continued to oscillate between confidence and anxiety.

9/15/85 Another great day in every respect. Philip and I are hiking along real smoothly. I feel great. It's good to get some excersize and I've really forgotten or feel fine about M and college. . . . Everything is going well. I feel self-confident, good. I slept real well. . . .

9/20 . . . One thing I do know is that I am really respected by a lot of people and I have to watch that because I can hurt them unintentionally. . . .

I made a list of colleges that I'd look at. Just the thought makes me anxious. . . . I can talk real positive and still feel insecure.

He reveals the discomfort he felt about the expectations of his AP history teacher in a letter to a friend.

They've always said at school that a historian's politics influence their interpretation, but in reality it literally controls their entire perception of an event. . . . History is the one class where I really feel out of place because everyone (including the teacher) is real conservative and proud of their fat bellys.

Around this time he began to think about whether he might be gay.

Sometimes I know I feel a little homophobic, like I'm afraid to be close to fellow males, even where there is little implication of sex, but of course there's often if not always a subtle underlining based on our sexuality. Convinced myself that I'm gay and might as well face up to it, but it isn't true wholly, by a long shot. . . .

In gym we've been talking about AIDS and I've been answering the questions. . . . a kid came up to me and started talking totally out of the blue. I've always thought he was gay. I gather he thought I might be gay. Am I? That is the question of the day!!!

Arthur hoped Aaron would go to MIT, where his father and sister had earned degrees. But Aaron didn't want to go to another large science school after four years at Stuyvesant.

"I think I'd like to go to Swarthmore," he told me as he looked over a heap of college catalogs. "It seems like a nice, small school. What should I do about MIT? I don't want to go there."

"I think you should apply," I said. "So Arthur feels you're considering it. He'll be upset if you don't. You don't have to go."

November 85 I had my MIT interview today . . . it was fun chewing the fat with this alum up at the exxon building. These interviews are actually kind of fun if you don't take them too seriously, but then one runs the risk of not getting in to college, and that would not be a lot of fun.

I have no doubt that the alum who interviewed Aaron also enjoyed their conversation. Whatever the worries Aaron recorded, with adults and peers he was poised, respectful, self-respecting, and abundantly intelligent.

12/1 After a totally unproductive, including shit, weekend, I sat back and spoke with Ingrid about Stasha, and Arthur, and history. I love to think about how things are different when Stasha is home and how things are different when she's away.

Its good to . . . try to figure out what fears are driving me. A fear of college and separation, and of doing badly in classes, and of not getting along with friends. That about covers it.

That fall I enrolled in a poetry workshop at City College with the poet William Matthews. Returning several poems, he suggested that their fragmented quality might come from my not believing that I was a good poet. I could be more expansive and write in complete sentences. This helped me counter my profound belief that nobody was likely to attend to what I said for more than a moment, so I had better pare my words to a minimum. His enthusiasm about my poems was heartening. For the first time someone I respected outside the narrow circle of my friends praised my writing.

The subway ride up to City College every Thursday afternoon became familiar—the moment the train rose out of its underground tunnel and ran elevated to the 125th Street station, then sank below the surface again to let me off at 137th Street. In class, Matthews folded his long frame into the seat at the head of the seminar table, presiding with an invisible cigarette in one hand and a drink in the other. The students formed one of those happy groups that sometimes comes together, generous and accepting and easygoing. My poems took on a stronger voice when I followed Matthews's advice. His continuing praise as I presented more work gave me courage, his words balm for the self-doubting soul. At my desk I struggled daily with my novel, now plowing through a second draft. In my poems I seemed to have a better sense of how to get myself on paper.

Tall, willowy Katherine, with brown hair flowing down her back and an open, smiling face, gradually became part of our lives that year. I had met her the previous spring as we prepared for a protest in Washington against US intervention in Nicaragua. Several of Aaron's friends stayed over the night before, so they could catch a bus to the demonstration leaving from nearby Union Square. They bumped around for what seemed to me half the night in the room right over our bedroom. When I made my disgruntled way upstairs at five in the morning, there was a youngster I had never met disarming me with a cheerful smile.

Katherine and Aaron went to more demonstrations. They hung out with Philip. "Stuyvesant had a lot of great students, but Aaron and Philip and I were the crème de la crème," Katherine boasted engagingly, years later. In Aaron's journal is a poem about their threesome, probably composed to the tune of one of his favorite songs, Suzanne Vega's "Tom's Diner."

> I am sitting in the subway
> With the three of us together
> And I love myself too much to
> Really give a holler
> And if life were really
> Simple I would eat some rice
> And beans.

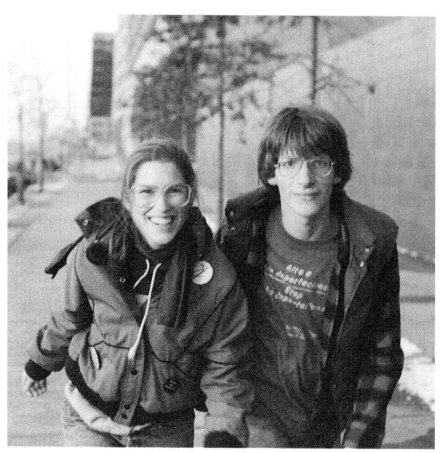

Katherine and Aaron, 1985

Why I don't know, but this was a period when Aaron did a great deal of tie-dying of his T-shirts and long underwear and regular underwear and sweatshirts. He embroidered an archipelago of patches onto his jeans, and another on Katherine's.

2/6/86 Tomorrow I go to MIT in order to visit. Oh blaah! . . . Had breakfast w/Katherine, that was sort of fun. I sit there being overwhelmed with love. . . . We're writing the book on asexual relationships, although I get sick of the topic sometimes.

He had begun attending meetings of the New York Nicaragua Construction Brigade, preparing to join a group building new houses in Nicaragua after his graduation.

2/10/86 I want to go to Nicaragua for the summer and have vague fantasies of spending a year down there if I could find some useful way to contribute to the whole shibang.

While Aaron was thinking of a visit to Nicaragua, I spent a week there with an artists' solidarity group. At a public meeting in the coffee-growing countryside, we sat in the scorching sun waiting for President Daniel Ortega, along with 2,500 campesinos and several veterans of the Abraham Lincoln Brigade. At last Ortega arrived and the campesinos could present their requests. The North American men—reporters and bringers of material aid—towered over them.

The women who guided our little group around the country, the representative we spoke to at the National Assembly, and the campesinos in the countryside were all caught up in the transformation that had altered their lives so dramatically. But as our van traveled the rural roads, groups of children often played by the wayside, their feet bare, their skin cracked with dryness, their noses runny, and their clothes ragged. Hardest to bear was the longing that came over their faces when they saw us in our sturdy sneakers, carrying bright daypacks and water bottles.

In New York I faced again the contrast between the wealthy elite, easily visible in the city's affluent neighborhoods and expensive restaurants, and the homeless people living in Tompkins Square, a block from our house, in a small village of makeshift tents and cardboard lean-tos. So I joined the Lower East Side Sister City Project, a solidarity group supporting the Nicaraguan city of Bluefields on the Atlantic Coast. We raised money, we shipped material aid, we ran a series of poetry readings.

When my parents were visiting, my father asked about my trip to Nicaragua. How can I describe the mix of love, exasperation, respect, and deep unease I felt for my father? Despite my ambivalence, I was happy to see his familiar face. There he sat on the living room couch, his long dark head with its strong features turned to me, his intelligent eyes expectant. Next to him was my plump mother, her short white hair waved in a neat bob. She looked nervous as he opened this dangerous topic.

I told him some of my impressions very briefly, knowing he didn't want to hear much. As a stalwart Cold Warrior, he had to disagree with me.

"I know you don't see it as I do," I said.

"You aren't objective. These revolutions always end up the same way."

"Daddy, I love you. You're important to me. But it gives me great pain that you do the things you do. I don't understand how you can." I was talking about his book on counterinsurgency policy and his commitment to the idea that the US should oppose Communist movements all over the globe.

"My book isn't a clarion call to action; it's an objective history," he said. He believed firmly in the objectivity of his own opinions and the subjectivity of mine, which were the result of my poor judgment and refusal to face facts—even, he would say when pressed, my gullibility at the hands of those who would dupe me.

"Your book has a point of view," I said.

"Yes, it does." Then we were silent. He was upset, I nearly in tears.

Both my father and I understood political issues as moral issues. I thought it wrong for the US to go around the world working to overthrow one government after another, from Iran in 1953 to Nicaragua in 1986. My father thought American interventions abroad were required by the crimes of Communists, who must be balked in their efforts to gain ground "by stealth and deception," as he said in his book on the Vietnam War. I thought there was plenty of stealth and deception in his own work at the CIA. And so our battle went.

5/14/86 Katherine came over and I felt a lot better. . . .

So after a bit I felt like it was OK to love her and lie on her, and be intimate and feel good or feel shitty with her and go to her for support.

So I told her all this and it felt better. We were sitting on this couch in the living room and we kissed and licked each other and hugged each other and felt each other being there and it was such a relief to love her and have a little trust that she didn't mind being loved and touched and adored. . . .

Katherine scrawled one of her many notes on notebook paper, probably in class:

Dearest Aaron,

I miss you more than anything. I want/need/would love to spend time with you more than anything. Just to hold you & be held by you—then everything would be okay.

Aaron loved and was influenced by Arthur. "We actually get along very well," he wrote in his journal. Still, he commented occasionally on his Oedipal feelings.

I'm writing mainly because I was sitting in the dining room with Ingrid, whose leg was on the table, and she took it off as Arthur opened the door, because maybe John was with him, and as Arthur came in and started talking I got this horrendous anxiety attack. He was talking about some rally he had been to.

Oedipus, good old Oedipus. I had an oedipal dream two nights ago. . . . I was masturbating and as usual at the very beginning everything is relaxed, but it tenses up pretty fast. Fear of hurting women, Oedipus complex, sexual orientation.

Remember: There is no reason confusion and wrestling with things should be bad. I have to have faith that I can figure it out.

Philip has been very sociable, intimate, friendly. . . . He's fallen in love. . . .

And undated:

Trying to respect myself. Desperately trying to respect myself. Desperatly. Desperatley trying to feel good about myself. Trying to be able to be at home with my body and with my sexuality. . . .

As spring approached Aaron told Arthur he didn't want to attend MIT.

Arthur got mad . . . He says if I have the ability to do theoretical physics I should, and I said yeah, and you should paint. He didn't like that much.

Aaron was referring to Arthur's degree in art and several years as a painter, which ended when he threw himself into leftist politics in 1968.

Sometimes Aaron complained of my irritating side:

10/6/85 Ingrid just came in and moaned because . . . I stopped the washing machine in the wrong place in its cycle . . . but then its possible that someone else did it, she says, in the most disbelieving tone, while my head starts to ache.

In essays for teachers, Aaron shows himself to be aware of his strengths and pleased with his successes.

On the whole I am proud of the situation that I have managed to put myself in at Stuyvesant, and knowing that I can do this makes the prospect of college a good one.

But I wonder how deep that optimism was, considering the uneasiness of the journals,

the fear of not being respected by my teachers, and not being able to be myself in any of my classes except English [with Frank McCourt] which is such a relief, an amazing relief.

In due course Swarthmore, Williams, MIT, and Oberlin accepted Aaron with letters cordially urging him to attend. His feelings were mixed. "I got into MIT and have to think about college (Oh boy)," he wrote, in a list of things that were bothering him, and then went on to complain about Arthur.

Arthur's here and I have a resistance to telling him how I feel and I find his attitude about all sorts of things unbearable from education, feelings (which he seems to think play too big a role in people's life and are a weakness, not a strength ie: being affected by the attitudes of the people around you) He asked me how I was and when I said I was OK he said "You are?" in the most disbelieving fashion. I know if I say something like I was upset because my friend was drunk and out of control, or that Stasha's rivalry (and mine) bothers me, that I would feel like he was slighting me.

In the end Aaron chose to go to Swarthmore. As he prepared for college, I was sad. But I didn't fear he would drift away. Perhaps because he was already so independent, our relationship didn't seem likely to change a great deal.

"I'll miss you. I'll be lonely when you're gone," I told him.

"I'm the one going away," he said, unhappily.

After graduation, he went with the Construction Brigade to work in the Nicaraguan countryside. Like Stasha, he had studied Spanish, so he would be able to communicate directly with people. Having been there so recently myself, I could imagine the dry landscape and the people he worked with. But it was worrying to listen to the news reports on the war, going on not far from where the brigade was building houses in Estelí.

On his return, Aaron was thin and proud of himself and increasingly reluctant to start at Swarthmore.

College is scary as all hell right now as I try to think what my relationship with fellow students is going to be like. I don't want shitty relationships, nor do I want to act superior and condescending.

Arthur and I were with Aaron at Naushon Island when he told us he had decided to defer Swarthmore until January. We had walked a couple of miles along the sandy trails and across fields of high grass thick with Lyme ticks, our pants tucked into our socks. Now we sat looking out towards Martha's Vineyard.

"I can drive a car and I can earn money—I don't want to go to college and be a freshman," Aaron said.

Upset by Aaron's decision, Arthur scolded him. "What are you going to do?"

"I can work with some of the *brigadistas* as a carpenter. Somebody's hiring a crew to do a renovation uptown."

Aaron's postponement of Swarthmore didn't bother me. After graduating from high school, I had put off college for a full year. And it had always struck me as a good idea for young people to have some time as civilians, knowing the world in another way than students do. Aaron would go on to do well at college, I had no doubt.

Like Arthur, my father was disappointed in Aaron's decision to delay Swarthmore. He irritated me by making scornful remarks about Aaron's job. He sent Aaron a book by a prominent Cuban counterrevolutionary describing the evils of Cuban Communism. Apparently he brought the book up with Aaron without making a dent in his views. Later he told me, "I had hoped Stasha and Aaron wouldn't grow up to agree with you and Arthur. It's a tribute to you that they do."

That was the kind of remark that made me love him. He revealed in one quiet sentence his awareness of his own fatherly failure to persuade me to see the world his way, and his recognition that the relationships Arthur and I had with our children were far different, as I had always intended.

———

As a small child Aaron had infuriated Stasha by insisting he knew everything. When he was older, she took it for granted that he did and took advantage of it. He went to Oberlin to help her buy a car, going to used car lots and looking under hoods. He could do anything on the computer, he could get the best deal on whatever he was buying, he could fix the vacuum cleaner, hang a shelf. We all turned to him.

Katherine tells a story of how she became aware of Aaron when they were taking health class together at Stuyvesant.

> For a few weeks we had a teacher whose classes consisted of lecturing us, don't smoke, don't have sex, if you have sex you'll get pregnant, that's terrible. After listening for a week or two I got fed up and I yelled at him, "You don't understand anything." He said to see him after class. So after class in the hall, instead of looking at me, he was looking over my shoulder. I turned around and Aaron was standing behind me. He said, "I agree with her, and whatever you have to say to her you can say to me too."

I shared Katherine's feeling: Aaron had your back. His intelligence and strength supported those around him. Once, when we were passing a piece of paper back and forth, writing notes, he drew a box on the page, and under it wrote:

This space for Ingridity.

I had been too young when my children were born, confused, self-centered, and volatile. Stasha had suffered, though I knew she was fundamentally sound. But Aaron had been able to use his abilities to leap into another sphere, into self-possession and ease. That last fall at home, he wrote:

So I came home from work feeling pretty OK. Same as usual.

Thinking I look beatiful. Proud of my car. Reading Invisible Man and liking it.

Working with Aaron's notebooks and school folders, I have had the pleasure of being with him day after day, of hearing his voice, and reading his sensible, intelligent essays. I've been happy that he enjoyed hiking with Philip; laughed and sighed over his hypochondria; been ruffled when I thought Miranda and later Katherine gave him a hard time. But his journals have revealed fears that I wasn't aware of, either because he often kept these feelings to himself, or more likely because when he did talk about them, his anxieties seemed pale next to his abilities and self-possession.

Chapter 6

As Aaron prepared for Swarthmore, he wrote to Katherine about his trepidations and inclination to withdraw.

> I'm afraid of being anti social. I feel like I avoid social situations, or that I will . . .and that I feel better about going to Swarthmore because I feel it will be easy to do that avoiding. . . . I shy away from group situations because I'm not sure I'd feel comfortable just being myself.

In January, not long after his nineteenth birthday, he set out for Swarthmore with Philip, who was already attending Haverford, also near Philadelphia. Arthur and I helped the two of them carry Aaron's things through the rain and slush on 9th Street to his Honda Accord, a venerable little car passed on by a cousin. They hopped in, one tall blond youngster on the left, the other on the right, and closed the doors. We stood sadly by the curb to wave as the car pulled away.

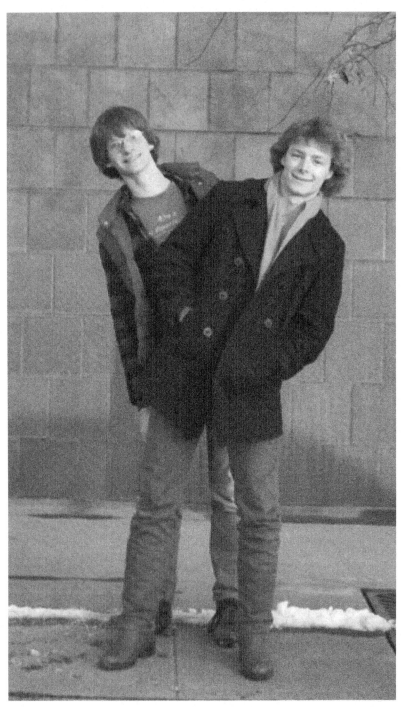

Philip and Aaron, 1985

Inside Arthur and I lay down on the couch to comfort each other. "Poor Arthur," I wrote in my journal. Poor Ingrid, I might have said. Now my days would be empty of Aaron, as well as Stasha. I would be alone in the apartment on Arthur's late evenings.

Aaron reported on the phone that he liked his physics. "We did $F = ma$ today," he said. "We talked about Einstein. Einstein thought that the universe was held together by its own structure rather than by force, or by the interactions between things in it."

A few days later he attended a protest against Eliot Abrams, a key figure in Reagan's war on the Sandinistas.

"How was it?" I asked.

"It was OK," he said. "There were about a hundred fifty people. Philip came over."

"Was it good to see him?"

"It was OK."

"How's your room?"

"Pretty good. One of the better things. The dorm is wood. I put up a notice on a bulletin board that I can repair bicycles."

Home over the weekend, he told me, "People at Swarthmore spend their time studying."

"But you're doing all right?" I asked.

"Except for about half an hour the first night. That was terrible. Not OK."

I understood this to mean that Aaron had had an anxiety attack. All too familiar with this form of misery myself, I knew such moods were disturbing but transitory.

Before long Aaron was talking about his new friend, Susanna, a philosophy major. For the two of them, it wasn't enough to take a full load of demanding courses. They went into Philadelphia every week to participate in a study group devoted to Marx's *Das Capital*.

Later Susanna wrote about Aaron:

> When we first spoke at Swarthmore . . . he had seen my name on the Nicaragua Construction Brigade's mailing list. We were the only students in the incoming class on that list, he pointed out. He was wearing his Sandino T-shirt. I always liked the way that shirt looked on him, slightly stretched across the chest. From the first moment I saw him I felt connected to him. He was quiet, understated and confident. He took daily life easily in stride. . . . [I]n large things and small, physics, carpentry, the arrangements of everyday life . . . Aaron was deliberate and directed.

In March I did a reading of my poems at the Poetry Society of America with students from several college poetry programs. Bill Matthews had asked me to represent City College. With much excitement I prepared, rehearsing my poems on my own and then with the coaching of my favorite cousin, Weslea.

To my surprise, as I stood at the lectern preparing to read, Aaron was sitting right in the middle of the audience, my beloved Aaron, smiling at me. Arthur sat further back. He had found a way to leave the *Militant* early, even though it was one of his long days. My friends were scattered through the audience, listening, reacting to my words. How good to have people who wanted to hear what I had to say, who appreciated my thoughts, my humor, my self, as I had managed to get that self into words.

On visiting weekend, Aaron showed us around Swarthmore with its well-kept lawns and attractive arboretum, and introduced us to his professors in the physics department. In the basement of his dorm, he showed us where he hid his food. He didn't like the dining room and wasn't allowed to store food in his room, so he had found a way to conceal a box of cereal in the ceiling of the basement storage area.

This didn't make sense to me. Breakfast is the one meal it's hard to mess up, even in a college cafeteria. That and his jokes about the college made me uneasy. His attitude was new—sneering and belittling, and unlike him. Yet at home for weekends every month or so, he was neither sneering nor odd, but as he had always been.

That summer Aaron again traveled to Nicaragua to work with the construction brigade, this time building houses in Morillo across Lake Nicaragua from Managua. Because of this work, he was asked in the fall to speak at a solidarity rally in Philadelphia, a memorial for Ben Linder, the young American volunteer shot by Contra soldiers a few months earlier.

Before the memorial Aaron showed me the speech he had drafted. Reading it, I saw that he was criticizing the way the brigade made decisions, which I knew would not sit well with the organizers of the rally.

"They aren't going to want you finding fault with the brigade at a solidarity event," I said. Aaron reacted as if I were attacking him. Immediately, I was upset with myself for being tactless.

On reading the speech, the rally organizers decided to make him last on the program. This meant he followed everyone important, and also the pitch for money, so that while he spoke people were beginning to leave, as usually happens as a long political program winds down. "And I changed the speech," he said on the phone. "I took out the part they didn't like. And at the end I said, 'Ben Linder! *Presente!*'" This was the formula used to commemorate the martyrs of the revolution, a conventional conclusion the organizers of the memorial would approve.

I knew it must have been awful for Aaron to be publicly embarrassed in such a way, put in a position where people turned their backs on him and walked away. And he was still upset with me for trying to warn him that the points he wanted to make wouldn't be welcome, as if my caution had caused his disturbing experience.

He withdrew from Swarthmore for the spring semester and found himself a carpentry job in Philadelphia, fabricating hospital nursing stations. He stayed on in the house he was sharing with other students in Wallingford, where he and Susanna had taken up residence the previous term. But Aaron no longer confided in me much about his romantic relationships, so I wasn't sure he was still close to her.

Was it around this time that Aaron told me, then told Stasha, then Arthur, that his sweat had such a terrible odor that he was uncomfortable in class? He was very disturbed. After consideration, I reasoned that it must have to do with late adolescent discomfort with his peers and with his body. He was anxious and this was the shape his anxiety took. What else could it be? None of us had ever found anything to notice about the way he smelled.

That summer Aaron traveled, first with Susanna, then Katherine, and then Arthur. He and Katherine wrote to Philip in June from New Mexico.

Hi. We're in New Mexico. . . . Susanna and I drove to Houston, where she stayed to catch a flight to Mexico, and I came along to Albuquerque and picked up K at the airport.

In the same letter Katherine wrote:

> Aaron looks "very gay" & sexy & available these days with
> a sexy tank-top and his ear cuff, not to mention his very
> baggy pants & size 40 hiking boots. So I'm thinking of pick-
> ing him up. Have you ever had him lick chocolate off your
> leg? . . . Well I must say, for looking gay, Aaron's in love with
> an enormous amount of women. I've counted five so far. I'm
> not sure why he's seeing me & Susanna if he's really in love
> with Sumathi. Does he talk about her to you?. . . He's . . .
> saying, I've never fallen in love with someone like I'm in love
> with Sumathi. He refuses to make his love known though. I
> think he enjoys this unrequited love from afar. . . .

From Albuquerque Aaron again wrote to Philip, revealing
his feelings about Swarthmore.

> I'm looking for work and maybe housing. Also thinking
> about transferring to the University of New Mexico. . . .
> Swarthmore doesn't have so much appeal. . . . it's where I
> really struggled an awful lot.

After spending time with Katherine, Aaron met Arthur and
they drove to Chaco Canyon to see the ruins of an Anasazi
center of kivas and towers and hike to the outlying pueblos. Yet
Arthur remembers Aaron's sardonic jokes at his expense. And
Aaron felt sick enough for them to go to the emergency room
in Kayenta, where the doctor found nothing amiss except perhaps some dehydration. Yet some of our best photographs of
Aaron come from this trip. In them he is smiling with an expression that is both sweet and proud, happy and relaxed.

When Aaron was home, I too thought he seemed gay, wan-

dering the city in his sandals and shorts, though I knew his relationships were always with women. He was nervous about
going back to classes at Swarthmore and consulted a psychiatrist
who prescribed an anti-anxiety medication. "It's the kind you
take just for the occasion. Actors take it for first nights. That

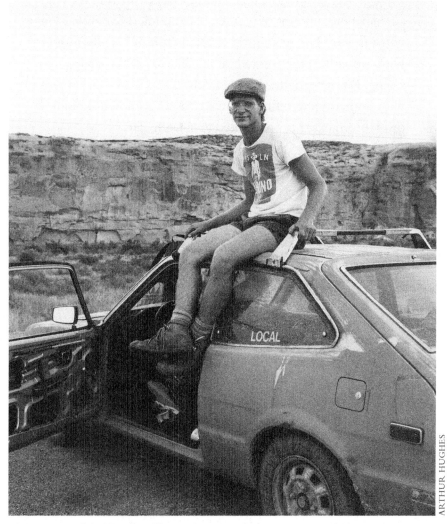

ARTHUR HUGHES

Aaron on his Honda, Chaco Canyon, New Mexico, 1988

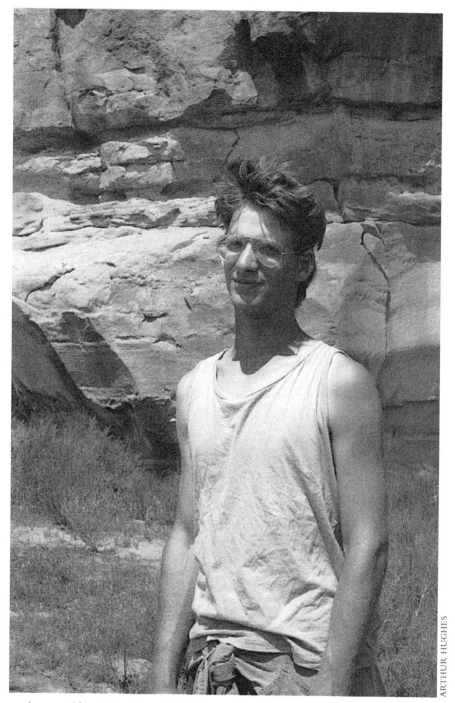

Aaron, Chaco Canyon, New Mexico, 1988

kind of thing," he said. "Just for the first few days of classes. She said it would be hard, going back."

At the end of August, Aaron again wrote Philip, who was in Bogotá for a semester.

> I think Susanna and I are breaking up. I'm not sure how to deal with the situation. . . . I mostly feel like if we kept seeing much of each other we would argue a lot, and things wouldn't work out, which is nothing I want to put myself through right now. Nor am I going to be doing much "political work" I think. It's time to be more adventurous and see what's out there. I think art or dance or theatre or something like that would be fun. . . . I'd like to have some technical proficiency in some section of the arts. . . . Maybe I'll see more of Sumathi.
>
> Actually, I'm scared shitless about going back to Philadelphia, but then the worst thing that could happen is that I'd be miserable. We'll see. I could see a shrink if things got bad. . . .

Aaron bravely returned to Swarthmore, attending classes despite his continual anticipation that others would be repulsed by his terrible smell.

He wrote Philip again in September:

> Everything is basically OK here and I'm having some success in doing what I want, which is to be a student at Swarthmore. . . . It's a bit like being a first year student and not acting like I'm half out the door all the time, but I already know a lot of people. . . .
>
> This is all not to say that things aren't difficult but I'm slowly beginning to feel more normal again and more a part of things, less spacey.

No more politics right now, or physics or math or science for that matter. Two humanities courses, art, and a sociology course and an intro psych course all of which are not bad, but not thrilling. At least I'm going to them and diligently doing the work, and getting to know the people in them. . . .

So it goes, gradually recovering from a lousy eight months.

Even during his lousy eight months, he stayed in touch with Philip, and talked of other friends: Michael Dorsch, Sumathi Sivapalasingam, Richard Williams. He was close to Susanna, and his relationship with her overlapped his intermittent relationship with Katherine. This may have been the cause of the arguments with Susanna that upset him.

I do remember, perhaps from this time, Aaron's bitterness as he complained about some misdeed of mine from his boyhood.

"You won't make that mistake when you have children," I said.

"I'm not having any children."

The intensity of his anger startled me. Why shouldn't he have children? He played with the kids of friends gently and told stories of children coming up to him in the park or on the subway to start a conversation. Later, when I thought more about whether he might be gay or bisexual, this remark came back to me.

When Aaron went back to physics in the spring, he studied quantum theory, statistical physics, and several-variable calculus. Again he excelled. He was friendly with Amy Bug, one of his physics teachers, often chatting with her after class. She wrote:

[Aaron's] sense of humor and sense of proportion made him wonderful to interact with. . . .

Aaron did an outstanding presentation of something known as the Renormalization Group, which is a rather advanced technique in statistical physics. He understood the principles completely, and did an elegant computer analysis to demonstrate how the ideas worked, and how one could produce "flows in parameter space" which would indicate where phase transitions occur.

John Bocce, the head of the Swarthmore physics department, in his letter recommending Aaron as a doctoral student described him as:

> the most promising theoretical physics student I have seen during my 24 years of teaching . . . He is intelligent, inquisitive, amazingly creative, and willing to persevere on any problem until he solves and understands it.
>
> He has always shown that rare ability to strip a problem of its difficulties, restate it in more understandable terms, quickly devise a solution method, and generate creative solutions. I remember with great joy and some awe the numerous complete, well-written, and well-presented problem solutions he worked out during all of his honors seminars and in the many discussions I have had with him on general relativity.

After graduating from Oberlin in 1989, Stasha spent a summer with Aaron in Philadelphia in a big house they shared with other young people. Aaron talked about his summer construction job and the people he was working with, laughing about how much alcohol they expected him to consume and how he avoided drinking more than he wanted to, his usual poised self. Stasha reported that he cooked a lot—brioche, corn pancakes, carrot cake. He was the kind, together brother she had come to turn to almost as if he, not she, were the older sibling. Seeing her grow more disheartened with each one of a series of uninspiring temporary jobs, he sat her down and gave her a little talk that was both gentle and accepting. "What's up, Stasha? You need to set a light under your butt," was the message.

Stasha rallied and in September flew off to Ecuador to work as a volunteer in an orphanage in Quayaquil, an industrial town on the Pacific coast. When she fell in love with an Ecuadorian, she extended her stay till January. On her return to New York, she landed a job at Catalyst for Women, a nonprofit that promoted women in the workplace. There her job was to maintain files on women working at corporate jobs in order to provide candidates for headhunters. She spent a lot of time contacting people to update records, sending off faxes, working at a computer. After she moved into a shared apartment on Prospect Park in Brooklyn, she visited 9th Street often, joking about her job, a pleasure to be with.

Aaron was still flirting with the arts, or maybe art history or even architecture. He talked about Kaori Kitao, who guided his tutorial in art history. Over one summer he studied architectural drawing at Columbia. For this course he and I drove back and forth several times over the Pulaski Skyway in New Jersey, a series of steel bridges and one of the first elevated highways, which connects the Holland Tunnel to the New Jersey Turnpike. My job was to use his camera to take photos of the steel work.

"That's what you want me to photograph? The name General Pulaski Skyway?"

"Yes. That's it." He glanced at me briefly, his face relaxed and playful, a characteristic look.

"Done," I said. Aaron took an exit into Newark and circled around to drive the skyway again, directing me to take more pictures. I enjoyed my task of photographing the highway that was the bane of anyone driving it.

Chapter 7

Reading my journals for this period, I am disappointed with my lack of comment on Stasha and Aaron. But I wasn't paying as much attention to them by now. I had fallen in love with Jay, a poet and teacher, a smart and erudite reader who lived in the world of literature, as I did. I had fallen, I had plummeted, I had plunged thirstily into love. We had met at Cummington Community for the Arts, where I had gone to work on my novel, *Greta Liebenbaum*, and he to write poems. We got to know each other by reading and discussing each other's poetry. Jay's comments were intelligent, his expression intense as his brown eyes scanned a poem, his large head still when he read them aloud to listen to them. Eight years younger than I, he was living near Boston then, teaching freshman English at Boston University.

The crisis of loving Jay threw me into the air, as if I were an acrobat swinging from the grip of one partner to the hands of another, never feeling altogether sure I would be in the right place to make the transition successfully. For a while I felt sure

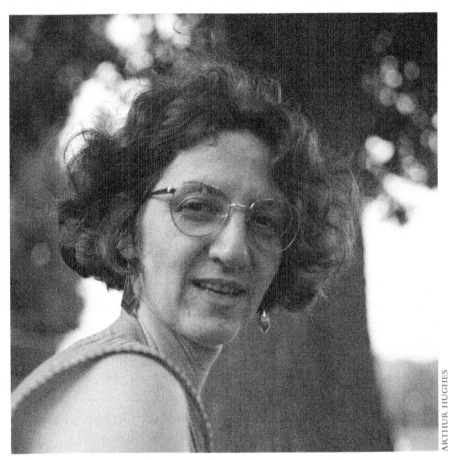

ARTHUR HUGHES

Ingrid, September, 1990

that my marriage would hold me securely and bring me back to Arthur every time. The flood of excitement and warmth I felt with Jay, the freedom to be spontaneous, silly, and lighthearted, passionate and serious, were more than I could resist. Why didn't I feel like that with Arthur? I don't know why, except that it has to do with the qualities of long-established love, deeply rooted and rich with years, but also constrained by habit.

I was reluctant to break my life apart before I finished the novel I had spent so many years writing. But as I got close to finishing, I thought about what would come next. Whether my novel was good, weak, or something in between, completion was an accomplishment. I would search for an agent, but I knew finding one might not be easy. Nor would publication guarantee success. I wasn't ready to start another novel, to embark on another stint in solitary. I wanted to continue writing—but I also wanted a new direction.

After almost two years of carrying on an exciting, trying, uncomfortable, secret relationship, I had to consider whether to leave Arthur. Why? Why did I want to undo my happy life? Why throw aside my solid marriage? I would like to be able to spit out a pithy reason for this. I've thought about it a lot. All I can say is that something in me chose to wrench myself willfully away from Arthur and start my life anew.

Work would be a necessity if I left Arthur. Though he had generously established a trust in my name years earlier, it didn't provide enough income to live on. For most of my life I had felt like an outsider, a feeling rooted in the dislocations of childhood. So I knew I didn't want a marginal position as a freelancer. I wanted an ordinary job, a job with a regular paycheck.

So I enrolled at Hunter College for a master's in teaching English to speakers of other languages. English was my medium, after all. It would be fun to teach adults, I thought. Having moved around the world so much as a youngster, I could identify with people grappling with a new language and culture. Teaching part-time would allow me to continue my writing.

At the end of my first semester at Hunter in the spring of 1990, I found my first job since college, as a tutor to ESL students in a summer program at Baruch College within walking distance of our house. Tutoring turned out to mean mostly that I acted as a classroom assistant to the teacher, a Chinese man whose first language was Mandarin and whose understanding of English grammar far exceeded mine.

During this time I printed out my novel. I took it to be copied, boxed it, and mailed it out to several agents. One was excited about it. I felt hopeful in a guarded way.

When I brought home my first tiny paycheck, I was almost dancing with pride. Then I steeled myself to talk to Arthur. On a warm summer evening, we sat facing each other across our dining table, as we had so many times. In his forties Arthur was fuller in the face than he had been in his youth, thicker in the waist, graying a little, still attractive.

"I have to tell you something," I said. With the jingle of a nearby ice cream truck playing over and over in the background, we began to talk. We talked for long, difficult months. Arthur's initial reaction wasn't anger or horror, but a deep sadness. For some time he slept little, trying to make sense of the past two years in his mind, sorting out what was happening and how he felt. We agreed to talk to a counselor but couldn't find one we liked in the middle of August, therapist vacation time. In September we met with Ellen Wachtel. As we talked more honestly, we grew closer.

That was the fall of 1990, Aaron's last year at Swarthmore. Yet he had decided to spend it at MIT as a non-matriculated student, studying quantum theory and working for an architect who was building his own house in Somerville. ("I've seen a lot of insulation in the last few days," he wrote Philip.) He was applying to several doctoral programs in physics.

"I like theoretical best," he told me. "But I'm applying in experimental."

"Why?" I asked.

"I think I have more chance of being accepted."

I wondered at his doubts. He had always gone straight for what he wanted. But I was hardly qualified to offer an opinion on the question of applying to graduate programs in physics.

———

Over the summer Jay had moved himself to New York from Boston. After a couple of months spent looking for work and living in a series of makeshift arrangements, just as the new school year was about to begin, he had an offer that appealed to him. It was a full-time job teaching in a basic education program for adults in downtown Brooklyn. He moved into an apartment in Brooklyn and brought his cat from Boston.

When I visited him, he talked enthusiastically about his teaching. Adults in need of basic education were a new student population for him, and he enjoyed teaching them. We talked also about my tutoring, books we read together, often facing each other at the table, so I was focused on his clear brown eyes and large, tawny head. (He looks like the Cowardly Lion in *The Wizard of Oz*, I told a friend.)

And then my mother learned she would have to undergo a heart operation to replace a faulty valve. The surgery would be at Johns Hopkins late in the fall. I could tell she was scared by the comforting tone she used to soothe herself and her stories of people who recovered from similar operations and a few weeks later were doing their rounds on the golf course.

I was scared too. It was a risky operation. But I didn't see how I could visit West Virginia, where my parents had lived since they retired. My own life was suspended in air, and I wasn't ready to talk about why with my parents. Instead of visiting, I phoned her often.

Suspended in air—and not entirely sure where I was going. While I was excited to be striking out on my own, throwing aside the habits of many years, I felt acutely the hurt I was causing Arthur and Stasha and Aaron. Plus uncertainty. How could

I know what happiness I might have if I stayed with Arthur, the person outside my siblings who had known me longest and best? Was I giving up too much? For the time being I was talking with Arthur, seeing Jay, feeling my way forward. How would I feel without Arthur? I still loved him—I knew that.

I had been hoping our sessions with Ellen Wachtel would provide a conclusive moment that would help me move ahead. When they didn't, I had one more session with my own therapist—how I would love to be able to say I made all my decisions without the guidance of a therapist—and told Arthur I was going to find myself an apartment and move out.

Yet I still wasn't completely sure I was making the right choice.

Aaron was in Brooklyn visiting Stasha when Arthur called them home to 9th Street to break the news. Half an hour later they were at the door: tall, slender Aaron and shorter, sturdy Stasha. Aaron leaned down and kissed my cheek. Stasha wrapped her arms around first me and then Arthur for a big hug, the kind you give when someone is in crisis.

"What's going on?" she asked me. "Daddy said you're leaving him."

"We're going to tell you," I said. "It's true."

We sat down at the heavy butcher-block table in the dining room. Just a few months earlier, Aaron had laid his hand on the massive table and said, "Things at home are really solid." Now I winced at the memory.

Today Arthur looked both sad and angry. Stasha and Aaron also were grave. "Arthur and I are separating," I said. Each time I used the word *separating*, which seemed to give more dignity to the process, I considered that it disguised the fact that I was the one walking away from our marriage. Arthur had made it clear to Stasha and Aaron that I was responsible even on the telephone earlier that morning. Still, it seemed kinder to say we were separating than that I was leaving him.

"Who is the man?" Stasha asked.

"Jay Klokker. You met him when you drove me up to Cummington."

"I remember. He's younger than you," she said, seeming upset.

"Yes. He is." I paused. "I'm not going to live with him. I want to be more independent. I'm going to look for an apartment and Daddy will stay here. We're considering selling the house." Stasha and Aaron knew my history, knew I had been twenty when Arthur and I married, and except for a few months before our marriage, had never lived on my own or supported myself. Arthur tried to talk but soon broke down. Aaron too began to cry, tears coursing down his face, his skin going red, his nose running. Stasha got up to hug Arthur, and I went to hold Aaron. When I released him, he rose and gave Arthur a hug too.

As we sat at the table, Aaron asked about selling the house.

"We have to get someone to look at it and tell us what it might be worth. It would help me to have my share of that," I said.

"You couldn't manage without that?"

"Maybe I could. I'll have to see. I have a little income from my trust, and I'm earning some too."

"We're thinking for now that I'll be here," Arthur said.

"Do you think it's impossible to work things out with Arthur?" Aaron asked me.

"I do think so. But we've been seeing a family therapist." Aaron looked even sadder. We talked a long time, until at last Arthur and Aaron went off to an exhibit at the Metropolitan Museum while Stash stayed with me.

"On the whole I'm proud of you," she said, speaking from her feminist side and thinking, I was sure, of what I had said about my need for independence.

I had known that telling Stasha and Aaron would be an ordeal, that they would be hurt and angry, that Aaron would be more disturbed than Stasha. I sat for a long time after she left, drained and dazed with tears, feeling as if I had been slogging through a snowstorm. This was the hardest time, I told myself. It wouldn't last forever. I shook myself and looked around. I was sitting on the couch in the living room—a good room, but like the rest of our apartment, it needed a coat of paint. Neither of us had been taking care of our house—symptomatic, I thought.

Aaron let himself in and joined me in the living room, settling himself on the other couch and extending his long legs in his jeans.

"Arthur went down to the *Militant*," he said when I asked. "What kind of relationship do you think you're going to have with him?"

"I count on him being my friend." I knew Arthur was unlikely to bear a grudge. He was a forgiving person.

"How is he going to get along now?"

"He'll get along. He has the SWP. He divides himself between the party and the family. He lets those two entities organize his time. I think he'll still do that." I spoke with the practiced glibness of an irritated wife. Was I a little condescending about what had seemed to me Arthur's way of distancing himself from my needs, or even those of Stasha and Aaron? Or was I mostly feeling anger beneath my analytic facade?

"He 'lets' them?" Aaron asked.

"He sets it up that way."

Now Aaron cried desolately, his face reddening again, his tears a flood, his misery my grief. "Arthur needs help," he said. "Without you who will help him?" He cried and cried while I went to get paper napkins to soak up his tears.

"Do you need help?" I asked after a minute.

"Yes. But I'm like Arthur. I can't make decisions easily and I don't know how to get help."

"Aaron, you can—"

"I don't need any blanket reassurances," he said. "I know it's possible to get help in the abstract." He reached out for me to embrace him. Kneeling by the couch, I put my arms around his broad shoulders.

"I thought you were doing OK. We've had a lot of good talks on the phone."

"If you think I'm OK and we've had good talks, I think I've been lying to you. I've been having such a hard time at MIT." His face was swollen from crying. "It's been so hard for me ever since I started at Swarthmore. There's so much discontinuity between me and you and Arthur. We're not like other families."

"What do you mean?"

"In other families the parents are both professionals. You and Arthur aren't like that."

"We didn't give you the models you needed."

"No."

"You feel like we didn't prepare you to deal with the world."

"Right." He was crying again, saying once more that we weren't like other families. I gave him another hug. It added to my distress to recognize his feelings, the feelings of my own youth, which I had tried so hard not to reproduce in him and Stasha. But Aaron sat up straight and blew his nose.

"Actually, I'm glad to have a chance to talk about the family." When he was calmer, he left for Stasha's. The two of them stopped over again the next day, sitting quietly in the living room with me and Arthur, grieving together.

I agreed with Aaron that Arthur and I were different from the parents of Aaron's friends. Who else had a parent who called himself a revolutionary Marxist? My writing wasn't such an unusual occupation. The mothers of two of Aaron's past girl-friends were writers—but their books were successfully published and mine was not. That was what disappointed him. My pride was hurt, but I knew Aaron was upset and that colored his feelings—about us and maybe even about Swarthmore and MIT. He had so many strengths. This would pass.

"You should have told Daddy when you first fell in love," Stasha told me angrily on the phone. I didn't contradict her.

"I'm going to get my life together. I made an appointment with my therapist," she said, referring to Ester Buchholz, who had helped her so much in her teens.

A few weeks later she greeted me at the door of her apartment on Prospect Park in Brooklyn, wearing the greens and aquas that suited her green eyes and thick, wheat-colored hair. I held her comforting plumpness to me. Since infancy she had had a kindliness I knew I could rely on.

We sat down to eat the lunch she had made.

"How are you doing?" I asked.

"I'm fine. I don't want to talk about how I feel." She spoke with a quiet firmness. Smarting a little, I found something else to talk about. I was glad to be with her, glad she wanted to be with me.

The four of us filed into Ellen Wachtel's office for our family session. Stasha and Aaron sat together on the couch; Arthur and I found seats in easy chairs.

Now Stasha voiced her anger. "I'm mad at Mom," she said. "She had a secret. I was trying to work on separating. But she already had."

Aaron was trying not to be angry. "I'm not blaming Ingrid," he said. But I knew he must be. The loss we all felt was my doing.

"You can get angry at your mother," Ellen said. "Were you close to your parents?" she asked Stasha and Aaron.

"Yes," Aaron said. Stasha nodded.

"What about Arthur? What's he going to do?" Aaron said.

"Your father will be all right," Ellen said. "I came to have a lot of respect for him over the months we were working together. He has a lot of strength."

"I guess it wasn't a very good marriage," Aaron said.

"Your parents did have a good marriage," Ellen said. "You and Stasha wouldn't be the way you are if they hadn't." She had said something similar to me and Arthur earlier. "There's mutual respect. And love."

"Yes," I had said at the time. "It's a lot to give up."

"It's a lot to give up," she had repeated.

But I did.

With Jay I shared the world of writing, and an ability to build a relationship as an adult, which I hadn't had when Arthur and I married. But Arthur and I could have started over with Ellen. He was willing to do that now. He had even been talking in the last months of returning to his artwork. That was something in his own control.

At a second family session with Ellen, Arthur, Stasha, and Aaron all voiced their anger. I knew this was natural and inevitable, but it was still tough.

Next time Aaron was home, he flared up again. When I commented on his anger, he began to cry. Later I was able to ask why he was so sad.

"I see no reason to be nice to you," he said with renewed anger.

"Because I'm leaving Arthur."

"Because you and Arthur are responsible for the way I am. You didn't give me what I need. I can't do what I want." He gave me a sore look.

"You can't? I thought you were doing what you want."

"I am. But it isn't easy. You didn't help me."

"I know I made mistakes. I know that. But we loved you so much. We helped you a lot. We sent you to good schools."

"You always let me make my own decisions."

He continued to berate me, leaving me baffled and worried. It didn't make sense to say he couldn't do what he wanted. He always had. He had made his choices with our support. We had provided him with what he needed. He had been so clear, as Philip said later.

Aaron's strengths far outweighed his distress. He had worked with a therapist for a time at Swarthmore; he knew therapy was a possibility, as he pointed out. One way or another, he would get through this bad patch.

Arthur was often out overnight now. He was seeing Lanie Fleischer, a woman we had known for many years. Capable, independent, a social worker at Rockefeller Hospital, she shared Arthur's politics and had been a member of the SWP for a period. When I had a chance I talked with him about Aaron.

"He was crying, and saying he can't do what he wants. Sobbing," I said.

"It's the result of your selfish indifference to the suffering of others," Arthur said, with an angry flash of his eyes. I couldn't dispute that I was being selfish.

"He feels unhappy at MIT. And he says we didn't bring him up well."

"He'll be OK. Of course, he can do what he wants." Like me, Arthur found it hard to understand Aaron's complaints. And he was distracted from Aaron's pain by his own. "You're soloing out of our marriage. I would never do this to you." He looked away now. I knew this was true.

"I'm sorry," I repeated, feeling how senseless and utterly inadequate it was to say this. How could my sorrow in any way make up for the loss he was feeling?

My mother told me she had prepared her plum puddings, as if she were making a promise to herself that two weeks after her operation she would be cooking Christmas dinner as usual, and Nora, David, and I and our families would all be together at the farm to eat it. My youngest brother, Billy, had been a Krishna devotee for twenty years, living in ashrams in India and Africa. Now he lived in California, struggling to support his children and rarely able to visit. After his decades abroad, we were accustomed to his absence.

As it turned out, my mother wasn't able to keep her promise to herself. While I was taking my finals at Hunter, she underwent many hours of surgery and suffered a stroke that swept away her ability to speak and paralyzed her right side. When I reached Johns Hopkins in Baltimore to sit by her bed, sometimes with my father, Nora, or David, she seemed as incapable as an infant and appalling in her unself-consciousness. She had been staid and proper and competent. Now she yawned with gaping mouth, picked at herself, allowed her fearful old body to be exposed when her gown slipped or the sheet worked down.

But she clearly recognized us, gazing at us with her brown eyes that were almost black, as mine are. By the end of December she had made enough progress to be on her way to a rehab hospital.

———

At home I began a new hunt when the apartment I was expecting fell through. Meanwhile, Aaron and I had a few peaceful days together. He returned to Swarthmore before I found a studio near Prospect Park in Brooklyn. As I packed my belongings and made arrangements to move, I came close to changing my mind. But I kept to my course, supported by the plan I had laid out, led by my intimacy with Jay. In the middle of February, I moved to Brooklyn, to a one-room apartment on the top floor of a walk-up with three tall windows looking out on a row of brownstones.

Chapter 8

In my new apartment I carefully arranged my desk and computer and books, the futon bed I had bought, a tiny table for cooking and eating, a bureau for my clothes. Though it was a tight fit, I brought a narrow day bed so that Aaron could stay the night with me when he visited New York. I felt I had fit myself into my new space tidily.

"It's like a boat," Jay said, agreeing with me. Here, I would live my new life of independence. In the corner with the stove and fridge, I cooked for myself, or Stasha or Aaron, who visited, though he never spent a night. Here I sat across the little Formica table from Jay, or we read to each other on the rose-colored futon. Sometimes we danced to Aretha Franklin. I wrote my assignments for my courses, had friends over to meet Jay.

Stasha brought salmon steaks and cooked for me my first weekend. She laughed as I showed her the glories of my tiny space.

"Look. There's a skylight over the bathtub."

"Look, there's a place for eggs in the fridge," she teased.

"It's a sad day," my father said when I called to give him my new number, a fairly mild way to scold me. But I felt chastened. I was shaky in my new life. Setting up the apartment had been the easy part.

For my father my decision to leave Arthur couldn't have come at a more difficult time. Despite his contempt for Arthur's politics and bitter shouting matches between the two of them, my father respected Arthur as a person and felt he was losing a friend. Knowing how burdened and sad my father was, I called often and visited when I could.

My relationship with my parents was rooted in the all-engulfing silence of my childhood. What I kept from them was an underwater continent, the continent of who I was. Only a few islands rose above the water: my polite self, my dutiful self. But these islands of duty and kindness and courtesy were what was needed while my mother was so ill. Planted on their firm ground, I let my political battles with my father go with a feeling that was almost relief. I didn't have to tell him what I thought of the first President Bush's Gulf War, declared while my mother was in rehab. He would always support American foreign policy.

I held my tongue even when I timed my visit to my mother with an antiwar protest in Lafayette Park across from the White House. "No blood for oil," I yelled enthusiastically, as I joined the crowd of protesters. Banners urged President Bush not to make war on Iraq over its invasion of Kuwait. It felt good to be with others who opposed the war, listening to speakers voice the outrage I felt over another senseless war.

At the rehab hospital I found my mother in the physical therapy room, sitting straight in her wheelchair, smiling and reaching out with her good arm as she caught sight of me. With the help of the therapist she was now able to walk. Her sense of propriety had been restored. She could follow what we said and she could read. But she couldn't produce language, either by speaking or writing. That was the hardest thing now.

In April Aaron drove me and Stasha to my parents' farm in the eastern panhandle of West Virginia. The winding road led through hills patched with woods and fields just turning green with this season's new grass. It was sweet to hear him and Stasha sing, "Country roads, take me home. . . ." The farm had been part of their lives since they were small children.

As Aaron pulled up at the farmhouse, my father came out to welcome us. Inside my mother was walking on her own, using her four-footed cane to help her balance. Her steps were almost like a toddler's stagger, so uneven I kept wondering if she would fall.

"Hi, Granma." Stasha and Aaron hugged her carefully, seeing how frail she was. The skin of her face hung loose, webbed with fine lines that had been plumped out when she had a good layer of flesh on her. But she was clearly glad to see us.

"Are you glad to be home, Mom?" I asked as we stood in the kitchen. She laughed, as if to say, that's a silly question. "Of course, you're glad to be home after five months away," I supplied. She nodded.

After supper my father talked about selling the farm. "I gave it to an agent," he said. "We've had a few people look at it already."

"You have?" I asked with some regret. I had known he was going to sell, but counted on it taking a long time.

"I've got my work cut out for me to clear out the attic. I need you to help me with that tomorrow, Ingrid."

"OK," I said reluctantly. What I really wanted was to sit in the living room and read a book. The large sunny rooms, decorated with the furniture and art and miscellany my parents had collected in their various postings around the world, seemed even more spacious after the confines of my little studio. I wanted to jog down the road through the woods to the Cacapon River and then take my time walking back up. I hadn't been able to keep up my running lately, with my courses at Hunter and work and moving.

When my mother was ready for bed, she rose and hugged us all again. Almost dying had swept away her old restraint, so painful and puzzling to me as a girl. My father followed her to the bedroom to help her with a devotion I never would have predicted, listening to my parents squabble. But now my father, despite his habit of assuming his needs came first, had organized his life around my mother.

In the kitchen the next morning, my mother came up to me for a kiss, her new, affectionate self. She had a way now of looking at you for as long as you would meet her gaze, like a child. Putting her thumb and forefinger to the corners of her mouth, she pulled it down at the corners to ask me why I was sad—she who had rarely asked me how I felt, who I had thought through all the years of my youth didn't care.

"I was just thinking that you'll be moving before long," I said. My mother nodded and looked a little sad herself. As my father appeared a minute later, her face lit up. Stasha and Aaron came in on his heels and helped me make breakfast. Then my father wandered off, while I lingered over another cup of coffee with my mother. Before long I heard my father bellow.

"Ingrid," he howled with an urgency I recognized, a combination of neediness and impatience I was capable of feeling myself. I rushed off to find him, so he wouldn't repeat his desperate call.

"What is it?" I asked, climbing the stairs. He was standing at the top of the pull-down steps to the attic, his head bent over a carton of old paperback books.

"I thought you were going to help me."

"I am. You don't have to yell that way. You'll upset Mom."

"She's used to it," he said, by way of excuse, and yet with a touch of humor. Of course, she was.

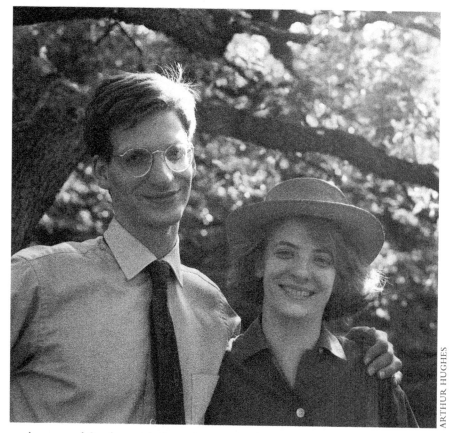

Aaron and Stasha at his Swarthmore graduation, 1991

———

After his graduation from Swarthmore, Aaron settled at Arthur's for the summer. When Stasha and Aaron, Arthur and I came together for my birthday dinner, Aaron was bitterly caustic. But when he and I made another trip to West Virginia, he was seemed well. He mentioned then that a research project supervisor at MIT had invited him to work on a particular project—but he had turned this offer down. Instead he would be teaching.

Visting him in Boston, in his apartment on Beacon Hill, I thought he seemed relaxed about his teaching and courses at MIT. He talked about a friend he was spending time with, and again the thought that he might be having a relationship with a man flickered through my mind, since this was the only friend he mentioned. In Brooklyn, I ran into Katherine on the street one day. She too had visited Aaron. "He seems kind of . . ." She made a vague gesture. "Kind of weird." But I knew he was doing well.

At Thanksgiving I loaded a turkey into a shopping cart and walked to Stasha's, happy the four of us would be together. In her large, sunny apartment, vacated by her roommates for the long weekend, the pumpkin pies Aaron had made were cooling on the kitchen table.

Soon Arthur arrived, dependable, easygoing Arthur in his gray workpants and gray parka, bearing the salad and the wine. To pass the wait once the turkey was in the oven, we went out to walk in Prospect Park. Stasha and Aaron posed for Arthur, arms around each other, smiling sweetly, Stasha in her black coat and Peruvian red felt hat, Aaron in a dark tweed jacket and muffler. I loved seeing the two of them together, knowing they had each other. Arthur was still central in my life, a charged figure, now in a new role.

Aaron seemed a bit uneasy. "Arthur the revolutionary," he said sarcastically, when Arthur referred to the Nicaraguan Sandinistas, now out of power. But Arthur wasn't easily hurt. Like me, he seemed happy to be here with Stasha and Aaron. He poured out glasses of red wine and said, "Cheers."

"To the family," Aaron and I said at the same moment. "And our achievements," Aaron added. Yet he seemed a bit moody. Was he sad about the family? I wondered. Was it his old separation anxiety? I hoped this gathering would reassure him that we were still a support for him.

"I get upset," I told Jay as we walked in the Brooklyn Botanic Garden. "Every time I get together with Arthur and Stasha and Aaron, it hurts." Jay looked hurt too when I said that.

"I feel so selfish," he said. "Wanting you for myself." He frowned down at me. I was silent. I was selfish too.

We passed the lusterless November green of the rhododendron hedges and followed the walk by the rose garden, the bushes cut back now for winter, until we reached the Cherry Esplanade, the wide lawn dry and brown, the cherry trees in their long rows bare against the gray sky, their glorious spring blossoms fallen months ago and swept away. Things wouldn't always be the way they were now, I told myself, as I had so many times in the past year.

We sat down on a bench, and to divert myself from my sadness, I asked Jay about his teaching.

"I have such a great group," he said. "They've taken over organizing our holiday party—all I have to do is bring paper plates."

———

Back in my little apartment on Carroll Street, I took two ibu-profen with a glass of milk and lay down. My head ached, so did my stomach, old complaints aggravated by the mammoth ad-justment of this time. It felt so natural to be with Stasha and Aaron and Arthur. I missed our foursome so deeply. Had I made a mistake? Should I go back to Arthur? But I didn't act. I didn't know how Arthur would feel now if I chose to churn up all the pain of the last year. He had his relationship with Lanie. Besides, I would hurt Jay and maybe hurt myself even more.

How great the price of leaving Arthur was. Beyond the ex-pense of training to be a teacher, of living on my own was the sense of being shorn of the strength and status, the security of a long marriage. Gone were sexy images of being a trapeze artist. I felt diminished.

At Jay's class party, the students had pushed their desks against the walls and were laying out big trays of food they had pre-pared at home. One was setting up the sound system for music. Jay welcomed me with a kiss and introduced me to the other teachers and his supervisors.

"You have a very energetic and talented teacher here," the program director said. Jay was buzzing happily around the room, accepting a gift from the class and saying a word of thanks, com-ing up to me now and then and kissing me. I marveled at his delight in his students, his freedom and spontaneity in the class-room.

———

"I can hardly get a word out of Aaron when I call," I told Arthur at our January lunch. He gave me a quick look from under his heavy eyebrows.

"I can't either. It's like talking to your internist when he gives you the lab reports. Perfunctory."

I thought Aaron was still angry over our separation. I bore primary responsibility, but Arthur couldn't avoid being tarnished too. In my preoccupation with my wrong-doing, my self-punitive thoughts, I was like a penitent who makes self-punishment a virtue. In fact it was more like a grandiosity, making me the center and the root of all that went wrong in the family and hindering my ability to recognize Aaron's developing crisis.

He visited me for breakfast one Sunday when he was in New York.

"What's going on with you?" I asked as he sat across from me at my little table.

"Nothing you can help with."

"But I want to help."

"I don't want support from anyone related to my childhood. I just want generic love from you and Arthur."

"We do support you," I said. "No matter what."

"You're too judgmental."

"I know I'm judgmental. I know. I've always felt bad about the time I criticized your speech for the Ben Linder memorial." Then, to my dismay, Aaron was sobbing heartily.

"That was a long time ago," I said.

"Four years," he said, holding up four fingers. Though I knew this incident had disturbed him, I was surprised to see him so very unhappy even now. When he was calm, we talked about other things a little. I persuaded him to see Ellen Wachtel with me the next time he was in New York.

I began our session: "Aaron seemed so upset last time I saw him. I'd like to be able to help him, to know what's going on with him."

"I don't want to tell Ingrid what I'm thinking."

"Why is that?" Ellen asked.

Aaron said again that Arthur and I had failed him, that we had never been successful. I had managed to let go of this complaint after he first made it a year earlier. It came as a new sorrow. This time I wouldn't be able to forget it. For now I could only sit listening to Aaron and Ellen. As she was wrapping up, I asked again if there was anything I could do.

"No," Aaron said.

"There's nothing you can do," Ellen agreed.

So I went sadly home to Brooklyn. Aaron was clearly not well, though I didn't know what was troubling him. When I met with Ellen again, she encouraged me to be matter-of-fact with him, to avoid bringing up emotional topics. She and I agreed that if he had a crisis, he would probably go to a counseling center or the MIT health service. I remember her suggesting I help Aaron hold himself together. I knew he was unhappy. I suppose I imagined a crisis might involve being overwhelmed by anxiety or feelings of inadequacy, feelings that had laid me low sometimes for months at a time. I didn't understand that Ellen thought a psychotic break was possible.

"His feelings for you are very complicated," Ellen said.

That didn't surprise me. While Aaron confided in me and retained some vestiges of respect for me, he was angry and unhappy with me at the same time. I was complicated. Why wouldn't his feelings for me be? These thoughts were not consoling. But there was no way to think about Aaron that didn't hurt. He wanted Arthur and me to keep our distance, a distance that by itself was a loss.

———

Then it was April and Aaron was on the telephone, telling me he was being taunted on the streets "in an organized and systematic way." Everything was changed. I was reeling. When I visited him in Boston, I found him a different person, his face contorted by feelings I couldn't guess at, his body as thin as it had been when he returned from Nicaragua at nineteen.

Now I can see how schizophrenia crept up on Aaron over the years. The bad first semester of sophomore year at Stuyvesant, when he was depressed, hypochondriacal, and often stayed home; the decision not to apply for a Westinghouse; the reluctance to start college may have been indicators. Especially about his experiences in high school, we can't be sure. Though hindsight can be useful in diagnosis, it can also make ordinary adolescent confusion suspect.

Philip saw a change, a sense of burden that began when Aaron started Swarthmore. Susanna wrote:

Early on in college he was certainly not the way he was in his last year. . . .

In that last year, he seemed much more burdened, more withdrawn. . . . Life seemed more of an effort. He was even more sardonic and sensitive to hypocrisy than I had known him to be. . . . He would mock anyone. . . .

Aaron himself dated the changes he experienced from the Ben Linder memorial in the fall of 1987. But it wasn't until four years later that he was plainly psychotic. The slow progress of his illness, the periods of remission in its early stages made it so we didn't recognize it until the stark truth lay before us.

Chapter 9

A few days after my visit with Aaron, he told me he had made an appointment with Dr. White, the psychiatrist whose name Arthur had obtained. I felt relieved, and relieved again a few weeks later when he began medication. He thought it was helping. "It makes things less extreme," he said. "I'm not so frightened by every little thing." When I spoke with White myself, he asked whether I thought Aaron might be suicidal.

"He's never said anything about suicide," I said. "In high school another student killed himself and Aaron was horrified."

"That's reassuring," White said. And then he said, "Aaron doesn't have to work with me, if you have someone else in mind."

"What do you know about the psychiatrist you suggested Aaron see?" I asked Arthur as we ate lunch at Veselka, the coffee shop where it seemed to me so much of my life happened.

"He's supposed to be easy to talk to. Good with young people."

I knew these were generic encouragements offered to recommend almost any therapist. "He seems rather young. And he didn't sound really confident," I said. But Arthur had been given White's name by a friend he respected and didn't consider my objections important. Besides, now that Aaron was seeing White, it would be disruptive to suggest he make an appointment with someone else. Still I continued to worry that perhaps White wasn't the best person to treat Aaron.

About suicide I didn't need reassurance, because it hadn't occurred to me that Aaron might consider it. But seeing him ill frightened me. My children were central in my life; their good sense and generous natures were part of me. Seeing Aaron sick and broken, not knowing what would happen next threw me into a disorienting uncertainty.

It wasn't long before Aaron was in New York for a weekend with Arthur, who had to work very late Aaron's first evening back. The phone woke me from a sound sleep around midnight. Arthur was calling from work, wanting me to phone Aaron, who was in the grip of his paranoia again. I sat up and turned on the light.

I could hear the anger in Aaron's voice as soon as he answered the phone. "What's going on?" I asked.

"You know perfectly well. As soon as I got back, just a little thing upset me. You know what it was. Whenever I get the littlest bit irritated with you or Arthur, you turn it back on me. You can't do that. No, no, no, no, no, no, *no*. You make it so I can't do anything. You might as well put me in a room and put a TV camera on me. You have to stop it. You have to stop."

"Stop what?" I asked, shivering, pulling the covers around me.

"You know. You *know.*" He went on ranting and repeating his accusations.

"Aaron, I know that part of you doesn't believe what you're saying," I said several times, as Ellen Wachtel had suggested.

"At this moment I do," he said each time. "You have to stop it. I can't do a thing without your interference. You know what you did. It's illegal!" His raving was repetitive and I wanted to hang up, but feared he would be upset if I did. Finally, in the face of my insistence that I didn't know what was happening to him, he said, "OK, I'll just have to pretend." We said good-bye.

The anxiety in my spine had landed full-force as we talked. I called Arthur to say he needed to return home. After a two-second debate with myself about whether to call White at midnight, I dialed his number. He was a doctor. This was an emergency. I got hold of him readily and explained the situation. A few minutes later he called me back. "I talked to Aaron. He's better now." I was able to relax a little.

Then a call from Arthur—he was home, Aaron was going to bed. I turned off the light and pulled up the covers as Aaron's words juddered in my head, preventing sleep. For now, according to White and then Arthur, his psychotic thinking had been calmed. How long the calm would last we couldn't know.

I was in a limbo of ignorance and numbness, alternating with the hope I never admitted to myself—that Aaron's psychosis would be short-lived. I think my shock protected me from fully reacting to what was happening—and now prevents me from remembering with any clarity. Much of this story, and almost all of the dialogue, comes from notes I made as events were unfolding, records of conversations I had entirely forgotten. Without my habit of journalizing, I would hardly have been able to write this book.

Once his dosage had been increased and had time to take effect, Aaron improved. We had long talks on the phone; he seemed to have forgotten his recent aversion to us. When I asked Dr. White Aaron's diagnosis, he said Aaron had a thought disorder. What was a thought disorder? I can no longer remember how I learned what this meant. Did Ellen Wachtel tell me that schizophrenia was described as a thought disorder and bipolar disease as a mood disorder? Or did I learn that later when I read more about mental illness?

I do remember reporting to her after my first visit to Boston. "He seems gay," I told her, thinking of his gait, which had the restricted quality seen sometimes in gays, especially in the days when they were so often confined to secrecy. She had evidently had the same thought.

"I wondered if the stress of keeping that secret might have been a factor in his breakdown," she said.

After his death I was able to get hold of Aaron's medical records. Then I learned he had told Dr. White that he began to fear rejection and to avoid other people after the Ben Linder memorial. His energy dropped. It hurt to read about his idea that he smelled so much he was repugnant to other students. He told Dr. White he had found "a huge amount of evidence" to indicate that "his body odor was offensive." He came to see it as a "smell of fear" that others could detect. Going to classes became painful, anxiety provoking." Finding it "impossible to proceed," he withdrew. Eventually, though he feared being discriminated against, he resolved to pursue the rest of his life. He told Dr. White: "Even though I smelled, I was still a normal functioning person. It was a handicap. But I went back to classes. I expected rejection all the time."

Despite Aaron's aversion to revealing the symptoms of his illness, so deep he hadn't been able to tell the therapist whose help he sought, he had told me and Stasha and Arthur of his terrible smell. I had made up an explanation, calling his idea late adolescent social anxiety. How easy it is now to be distressed by the gap between our understanding of him and his experience. But our perceptions made sense at the time. We couldn't imagine that our stellar Aaron could be in serious trouble. Even if Aaron had been a youngster who found school and relationships more difficult, we would have failed to catch on. His downs and ups would have seemed like an ordinary adolescence. Mental illness was not something we were equipped to recognize. Our ignorance blinded us.

Since the shame and embarrassment of the Ben Linder memorial, Aaron reported to White, he had suffered periods of deep depression. He called himself worthless:

"I was never one of the worthies. I was one of the misunderstood. I wasn't recognized. I was always afraid people wouldn't like me."

His description of himself contradicts his own high school journals and his academic record. But by the time he met with Dr. White, his illness had eaten away his understanding so deeply that he saw no honor in the As and the awards, in graduating Phi Beta Kappa, and being accepted at MIT.

Now he was watched in his apartment and imitated by people in the laundromat and on the street. Circumstances were arranged to see how he would respond. Someone, or a number of someones, knew "in glorious detail" things about his life that "no one should know."

White thought Aaron had been preoccupied with his delusions for a year and a half. A year and a half earlier was the start of the semester he spent at MIT preceding his final semester at Swarthmore. So MIT, or his feelings about being there, must have been the factor precipitating his delusions and later his full-blown psychosis.

The Forbeses had become for him an omnipotent force. It's true that Arthur's Forbes cousins call themselves part of the Boston aristocracy, in the same league as the more famous Lowells and Cabots and Lodges. It's also true that J.M. Forbes & Co. manage the investments of members of the family, and that JMF, as we called the firm, supplied Aaron with funds from his grandmother. Building on these real pieces, Aaron saw the hand of the Forbeses "everywhere. Professors were treating me preferentially." This seemed to have been a positive feeling during his first semester at MIT. But it had turned negative.

White described Aaron as "neatly dressed, no bizarre mannerisms or behavior, mood was anxious." He told White he was depressed but not suicidal. But he

> began to feel less in common with others
> in pain & no one knew
> felt others were rejecting me
> didn't regard anyone being able to understand
> deep hurt was being perpetuated
> didn't know how to organize
> brutal game trying to alter my behavior

Most wrenching for me, reading White's notes, is seeing how alone Aaron was with his "deep hurt."

———

In West Virginia my mother had suffered more strokes. My father insisted on treating her bouts of pneumonia aggressively, though she could no longer walk or eat, and subsisted on liquid nutrition given through a feeding tube. She shuttled from home to hospital to nursing home. At the end of May my father asked me to visit for the third or fourth time in the last months.

I called Aaron to say I was heading to West Virginia. "Granma is very sick," I told him.

"Maybe this time she'll die."

I might have considered this tactless, if it hadn't been such a long, miserable time that she'd been sick. It was horrible watching her diminish as one small stroke followed another, each one sloughing away more flesh, strength, hope. To get through this ordeal I suppressed my feelings as much as I could.

Lying in the white hospital bed, my mother would meet my eyes each morning when I came in. I would struggle to find something to say to her, then sit on the bed and hold her hand while I read my book. When the nurses sent me out of the room, I would sit in the cafeteria with a cup of coffee. Away from her during these breaks, I had a sense that I was fulfilling a responsibility that was almost a rite of passage, caring for a parent who was leaving life behind—or being left helplessly behind by life.

I missed Nora and David. Living in the Washington area a couple of hours away, they could have lent their support to my parents more easily than I could. But they were on the outs with my father. His chronic needling and insults had been capped recently by a dispute about the tiny cottage he had invited them to build in his back pasture. Their visits were rare now. For me being here was part of my love for my parents. Whatever their failings, they had loved us as well as they could. Their history was my history; their substance was my substance, and I couldn't turn away from that.

Driving west on Route 50 toward the end of the day, I would enjoy the luxuriant May greenery. The trees were fully leafed out and the blossoms had fallen in the apple orchards, where the trees were lined up in orderly rows. The high grass in the fields would soon be ready for mowing. As I slowed down for the little gravel road that led to my parents' farm, I rolled down the window to let in the spring air.

After supper my father would park himself on the couch to nod off, while I went to the bookcases where my parents' books stood, familiar in the way of elderly aunts you've seen since childhood at family parties. Searching my mother's collection of Trollope, I found one I hadn't read, *Doctor Thorne*. Stretched out on the couch, I left behind my parents and my absent siblings, Jay and Stasha, Arthur and Aaron, and let the world of Barchester envelop me, its aristocracy with their snobbery and pretensions, its good-hearted, handsome squire's son, its saucy, witty heroine, and its guaranteed happy ending.

As the days went by, my father became increasingly irritated with me and I with him. He objected to my efforts to find a practical nurse, undertaken because the hospital wouldn't release my mother until we had one. I thought I was being helpful, but he told me scornfully that I didn't know anything about some aspect of my mother's care. I lost patience and raised my voice.

"So I made a mistake," I said. "You insulted me."

He said nothing for a moment, then sat down across the living room from me. "I think you should exercise your judgment not to be so bossy," he said. "It gets my back up. Your mother would never do that."

"I'm not my mother," I said. To me her attitude had seemed part of her emotional absence.

"It's not too late to change," my father said. I held my tongue. I like having ideas and opinions and freely confess to being full of suggestions and likely to offer them up.

"Besides, I'm a touch depressed, and everyone knows that when you're depressed you tend to flare up." If that was it, he had been depressed all his life. His angry outbursts were part of why my siblings were avoiding him.

Seeing it was time to stroke my father a bit, I made a little speech about how wonderful he had been with my mother since her stroke.

"Thank you for your kind words," he said. He was a diplomat; I was his daughter. We both knew well how to produce gracious words, and perhaps also how to discount them. Even while I told him honestly I was impressed with his devotion to my mother, I preferred the distance of being irritated with him. Most of the time he made that easy. Still, our conversation was a marker of the greater intimacy that came with sharing this difficult time, allowing more of the submerged continent of Ingrid above water.

At the bus station the next day, my father said, "You're the best daughter in the world. I appreciate all your support. And how smart you are." I gave him a kiss. Despite discounting his statement as much as I had my own the day before, despite my deep ambivalence toward him, he was one of the anchors of my life.

Aaron sent me a gift of two hand-thrown demitasse cups and saucers. He sounded well on the phone. As he prepared for a weekend at Naushon with Arthur and Stasha, he asked if I

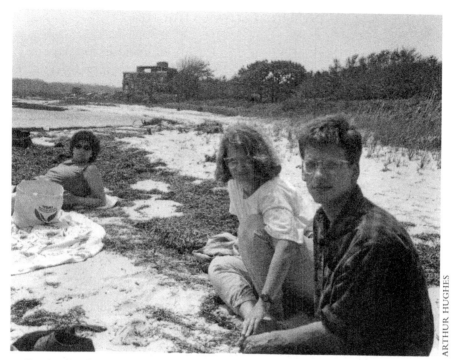

Lanie, Stasha, and Aaron, Naushon Island, 1992

would go too. It was painful to turn down his request—but I couldn't undo the past. I could ask him to visit my parents with me and Stasha, an invitation he accepted.

Stasha and I drove across the rolling green fields of Pennsylvania, Maryland, and finally Virginia, heading for Winchester, where we would meet Aaron. As we drove, Stasha squealed with anxiety. "Mom, the way you drive!"

She was a good driver, and I was happy for her to take the wheel, but that didn't calm her. "Why do they have the gearshift on the steering column? I'm used to having it at my side." "Can you actually see when you look over your left shoulder?" I was disconcerted by her attitude toward driving. But Aaron's illness had undermined her confidence in herself and made her world a more frightening place.

Much later she talked about Aaron.

When I think of Aaron, I just think of wanting to take a nap with him. We would be driving somewhere and I would bend one way and he would bend the other and we would go to sleep. At Ojai, where my grandmother lived, we would go for a hike up a sunny hill. And we would stop and take a nap. I would doze off on his legs. We did that more than once.

He was Aaron. He was always there. He was someone you take for granted. You could just be with Aaron. You didn't have to be anything. It's very rarely that you find someone like that. He was at ease. He was calm. He knew me so well.

Stasha had lost that closeness she didn't have to think about, the person she could trust so deeply. Aaron might recover, or he might not. Either way, his breakdown posed a threat: if this could happen to him, it could happen to her too.

Aaron stepped down from the bus looking like himself again. His jaw no longer bulged, he had gained back a little weight, and he was no longer grimacing. He hugged us both and seemed glad to see Stasha, though she was prickly.

At my parents' house, my father was making supper. My mother spent most of her time in bed now, in the bedroom suite off the living room, cared for with great kindness by Tammy and Rhonda in alternation, cared for in ways I wasn't sure I would have been capable of. Life was gradually deserting her wasted body. You couldn't look at her without thinking of death.

After supper we sat on the deck, looking rather sadly down the slope of the lawn to the gardens. I took a mental photograph of the roses and the fruit trees, the two barns, and the woods. This might be our last visit to the farm. My father had a buyer at last. In a few months, he would be moving himself and my mother into Winchester.

He walked up the slope toward us, his head down, his khakis hanging baggily, looking more stooped than usual. Dropping into a chair, he addressed Aaron. "The deck is holding up," he said. Several years ago the two of them had worked together to expand the deck and build a little gazebo in its corner. "I remember when you left, and I asked you how much lumber you thought I would need to finish up. It was the spot there, where the planks had to be cut at an angle. And you said, 'That's easy, Granpa. All you have to do is measure the distance and multiply it by the square root of minus one.'" My father threw back his head and laughed.

When Aaron had visited a year earlier, my mother had been walking with a cane, feeding herself, reading, alert, and responsive. Now when Tammy brought her out to the deck, she listed in her wheelchair, her head falling forward and to the side on the broken stalk of her neck.

"Mom, Aaron is here," I said.

She raised her eyes to look at him, standing by her wheelchair. Aaron was so appalled he laughed. Perhaps he saw her as an object lesson—this is what they can do to you, the ones who conspire against you. Or perhaps his laugh was no more than the kind of inappropriate response so characteristic of those living with mental illness. What my poor mother thought when he laughed I hated to think.

An old stone house on a quiet country road outside of New Paltz in the Hudson Valley was Jay's and mine that summer. I often sat on the flagstones outside the house, watching the wind bend the long grasses in the marshy fields and set the branches of the trees tossing. I wanted to write about how my parents seemed transformed in the last year or two, but I found it hard to concentrate. When I thought of my mother, I heard my own voice saying, Hi, Mom. That greeting she could never answer rang in my mind, as if it could conjure up her voice. Or as if it were a death knell. Night after night I dreamed of an endless cleanup following a family party, of chores that were never done, of trying to make order in a place that was always gloomy and dark. I would wake myself just to be free of it.

Jay hung his binoculars around his neck when we went for a walk, his quick eyes spotting a fossil in a rock by the road, or identifying a bird that was no more than a blur of movement to me. Most of the time he sat at his computer, chugging through a first draft of a clever time travel novel. His ability to transplant himself from one situation to the next made me marvel. In his various sublets in New York, in our summer rental, he quickly adapted. In a recent poem he compared himself to a hermit crab, a crustacean that adopts the abandoned shell of other sea creatures to protect itself, lacking one of its own.

In one of our phone talks, Dr. White asked me, "What am I looking for? What was Aaron like when he was well?"

"He was lovely," I said. "Charming, sensible, good at everything."

"I'm seeing that now," White said.

"But he doesn't understand that he was delusional. Doesn't he need to know that?"

"Not necessarily. In my experience, people often recover without that."

This increased my doubts about White. In my own therapy,

insight had been important: recognizing the fallacies that shaped my understanding had been part of getting over them.

In August Aaron told me White had agreed he could try going off his medication, although White's records show Aaron had never taken it more than intermittently. White soon found him preoccupied with his belief that the Forbes family was shaping his life. He believed now that he had been accepted into the MIT physics department as a Forbes, rather than for his own abilities. He became more depressed and reported that he was being followed and harassed, spied on by the Forbeses, who must have examined his belongings to know his business so well.

White noted: " . . . very little opening for self-observation or insight. Appeared thoroughly convinced of veracity of his experience." And he no longer trusted White, who was too "interested in Forbes" family. In addition, Aaron was "highly skeptical re meds. How will it help. Felt he wanted to directly confront problem . . . to go out and try to get a job and see if 'they' interfere."

Why had Aaron turned against medication? He never gave a reason, so I can only surmise that side effects bothered him: the dulling of the ability to think; dry mouth and constipation, the latter an old complaint of Aaron's. And if his problems were caused by people who interfered in his life, medication would be useless.

Aaron had been so much better over the summer. But as his fall semester at MIT loomed, he was calling me and Arthur and denouncing us belligerently. Again I went to Boston. He seemed happy to see me, ate the remnants of my lunch, said where he wanted to have dinner, and talked cheerfully about doing something we both liked the next day.

Next morning we wandered the site of the Battle of Bunker Hill, reading the historic markers and enjoying the sunny day. On the Boston Tea Party ship, a tour guide called the attention of his group to something in our direction, and everyone looked our way. Aaron insisted we go back to his apartment, where he turned and closed the door before I could follow him in.

On the train home, I gazed out the window in a funk, noting each time we crossed another river I couldn't name. To comfort myself I thought about what good friends Aaron and I had always been. I recalled meeting him one day as I crossed Third Avenue and stopping to give him a hug. An older woman had noticed us, and exercising her inalienable right as a New Yorker to kibitz on the action around her, said, "That was a good hug." There was some consolation in remembering a closeness that had been strong and happy and a stranger's witness, but the past couldn't tell me where I was now or how to go forward. I had scant understanding of the barren wilderness where I had landed or the angry creature with distorted features who was my own son. In the past Aaron would have been my support in getting through such an ordeal. Now he was the ordeal. Why had he sent me home? Though I had observed the tour guide pointing toward us, I didn't understand Aaron's thinking enough to know why he had turned hostile. What should we do now? I stumbled from day to day, not daring to think what might come next. Yet when I picked up a book on schizophrenia at the library, I read the first page and put it down again, still unready to learn about Aaron's illness.

Opening my mail I found yet another letter saying that my novel didn't suit, didn't seem marketable, or for some other bland reason didn't make the cut. I dropped the letter into a file and pushed the heavy drawer until it closed of its own weight. Probably I should revise the novel again, I thought. But though

I was sad, in all the tumult of that time, *Greta Liebenbaum* didn't seem as important as it had when my writing was at the center of my life. Still I continued to write and send out poems and stories. In fact, I was excited that a glossy magazine, *Lilith*, had accepted my story retelling the Biblical tale of Tamar.

Fall semester was my last at Hunter; I would graduate in January. The first of my student teaching assignments was in a fourth grade in a public school on the Lower East Side. Evenings I attended my own classes. Weekends were for everything else—taking the National Teachers Exam, writing papers, spending time with Jay or Stasha. I thought about Aaron as I rode the subway, walked the streets of Manhattan and Brooklyn, gazed around my studio apartment at my shelves of books and desk, heaped with work for my classes, bills, journals. I thought of Aaron as he had been before his illness, of the worrying paranoia that had him in its hold.

Aaron continued at MIT, still teaching his lab section, as his condition got worse and worse. He made derisive remarks about White.

"I'm dealing with the usual garbage. People say things about me in class," he said.

"Are you hearing voices?" I asked with a surge of anxiety.

He paused. "I hear people talking. Words come out of their mouths. They have harsh voices."

"Are you sure you're not hearing voices?"

"I just don't know how to deal with the locals. I hate people here. They don't know what they're talking about."

"Aaron, you need to take your medication. Then you could deal with the situation at MIT."

"It's not a situation. And I'm perfectly justified in my feeling about MIT. I just wish I could do something. What gesture can I make to show them that they're loathed and utterly despised? I want revenge."

"If you would take your medication, you would feel a lot better." I clung to the only possibility I saw for improvement.

"I'm taking medication."

"I don't believe you."

"Why?"

"You don't talk this way when you're taking it."

"Oh," he said under his breath. "I messed up."

I hung up and sat without moving for a long time. Aaron was hearing voices; he wasn't taking his medication. My urgings that he resume were born of despair rather than hope. It was six months now since we had become aware of his breakdown. He wasn't getting better.

For me this was a time of pervasive anxiety, headaches, and self-punitive thoughts. When Jay was visiting my little apartment, I told him what Aaron had said. But I didn't know how to take strength from him.

Seeing Ellen Wachtel with Arthur, seeing Arthur and the psychiatrist Ellen had referred us to, seeing Arthur and Stasha, talking to him often on the phone about Aaron's condition kept my regrets over leaving him active. I needed his cooperation, and it was forthcoming. I knew how deeply he loved Aaron, that he would help Aaron however he could. I continued to dwell on whether it was too late to go back to him. Even when it was far, far too late I maintained this train of thought, undermining myself more, eroding my pleasure in Jay, which was the part of my life that could have been happy. Keeping all of this to myself as much as I could, I kept putting one foot in front of the other.

Arthur, for his part, continued to see Lanie, and to share his political work with her. In the period of reevaluation caused by my leaving him, he had resigned from full membership in the Socialist Workers Party and assumed a less demanding role. He had taken up his photography again. The laundry room at 311 had become his darkroom, where he printed photos of the California mountains around his mother's house and of Naushon.

I drove up to my parents' farm on a mild fall day to witness the auction of those items my father had left behind when he moved himself and my mother to Winchester a few days earlier. Cars and pickups were parked along the lane and in the front field. A crowd stood around the auctioneer on the front lawn. From the sidelines I talked with Rhonda, who had been taking care of my mother for so long, and with Dossie Friar, a neighbor and recent widow whose husband had been a colleague of my father's. Like my mother, Dossie was English, and my mother had often talked of her, adopted her Christmas pudding recipe, and held her in high regard. Dossie was more inquisitive than my mother had been, asking me about my separation from Arthur and my children.

When the auction was over and people were loading their purchases into their cars and pickups and driving off, I found my father, always easy to pick out among others because of his height.

"Come on, Daddy. Let's split this two-bit taco joint," I said, recycling a joke that Stasha and Aaron and I liked. My father stared for a moment and laughed, as much with surprise as with amusement. He wasn't used to me being silly.

"I gotta get my money, honey," he retorted, equally uncharacteristically. So I headed to the hospital to see my mother, leaving him to follow when he had wrapped up.

At the door to my mother's room, a doctor I had never met was talking to a nurse. "She's in a coma," he told me. "It's time to talk about her living will."

"My father will be here soon." My mother lay as if asleep, her white hair cropped very short, her body so slight under the white covers that it looked like a child's. Putting my hand on her head, I felt the warmth of her skull. She was breathing peacefully.

When my father came in, the doctor explained again. My mother's condition was grave. The conditions of her living will had been met. She wasn't going to recover. What did we want to do?

"I want you to fight like hell," my father said.

At the idea of prolonging this misery for another cycle, I burst into tears. "I don't want her to suffer anymore," I said. I didn't want to suffer any more myself, I didn't say.

"She isn't suffering," the doctor said.

I hoped the end would come soon. She was such a thin remnant of herself. Her eyes, when they were open, had held the trickle of life that was left of her. Now they were closed.

My father had taken a small house on the outskirts of Winchester. That night I told him of Aaron's breakdown, his diagnosis of schizophrenia. Keeping it from him had become a burden, and I had decided as I planned my visit to end my pretense that everything was fine. If my mother's life was to go on in this dwindling way, as the doctor said it could, and as my father wanted, I might as well tell him now. He was disturbed, of course—even frightened.

I was in Brooklyn when the call I had been expecting for months finally came. My mother was dead. "It's hard," my father said. I knew that for him it was a harsh blow. As long as she had been breathing, he had felt she was there for him, knew him, loved him.

"It was a cruel death," he said when I reached him. I could only agree, though I believed it would have been less cruel to have let one of her many bouts of pneumonia carry her away. At least I had learned from her illness and death what to avoid for myself. My family would know my wishes well before the end was near. Already I had begun telling Jay and Stasha that I would never want my life prolonged by treatments that were painful and ineffective.

For me my mother's death was a release from the drawn-out dying-by-inches of the last two years. This would be the last trip for a while. I wouldn't have to find a way to get to West Virginia every month or two, with each trip adding another couple of hundred dollars to my growing indebtedness to Chemical Bank. One part of my burden had lifted.

It was comforting to spend the week calling friends and family, to help my father arrange the memorial and the luncheon to follow. It was so simple to be a good daughter—all I had to do was show up.

At the buffet after the memorial, attended by all three of my siblings, and my parents' many friends and neighbors, I found myself scanning the room for my mother. She had always loved to give a party. I missed her smiling presence, plump, dressed in patterned silk with a jade brooch, well coifed, enjoying the food and wine, talking happily with her guests.

My father's sister, Phyllis, and her husband, Buddy, drove me and Jay and Stasha back to New York after my mother's memorial. My uncle warned me, "Don't be surprised if your father remarries soon." I took note of his prediction as we drove across the rolling fields that were now a faded straw color, back to my square room with its three windows, back to the hallways and classrooms of Seward Park High School on the Lower East Side, where I was student teaching for the next month, back to dealing with Aaron's illness.

The next weekend I traveled to Boston again; Arthur and I had set up a meeting with Dr. White. Aaron opened his apartment door to me, and I handed him a bag of bread and cheese for our lunch. Putting it aside for a moment, he leaned over the table and with his large hand brushed away crumbs with a series of strokes I had often seen him make, a rapid, efficient sweep. Later I came back to that gesture, as if keeping it in mind would bring back competent, straightforward Aaron.

Feeling that his only hope lay in taking antipsychotics, which depended on his acceptance of his condition, I tried to convince him that he had a mental illness. (Was this a good approach? No. Had it worked so far? No. Did that stop me? No. Because no, I didn't know of any other approach.)

"After you started graduate school at MIT—"

"Now there's a sure sign of psychosis," he interrupted. "Going to MIT." So I had to laugh. As we continued talking, he asked me, "What do you do if you can't have what you want?"

"Then you have to adjust," I said, feeling how cruel my answer was. I knew he wanted to stay at MIT and doubted he would be able to. This hurt me. It had to hurt him even more. He had been able to attend any university, any graduate program he applied to, to do well at anything he was interested in. The times of his easy ability, of friends and many interests, were past. Isolated and under siege, his face reflected his tension. But he was dressed in clean denims and a sweater; his hair was washed and falling across his forehead. Though he had been missing his appointments, he had agreed to join me and Arthur today when we met with Dr. White.

He took a seat in the waiting area while Arthur and I introduced ourselves to White. In his office we spoke for some time of how ill Aaron seemed, how upset we were.

"He's hallucinating," I said. "He talks about things people say about him in class. He's not taking his medication. Is there any way you can get him on it again?"

"I can have him go for testing of his blood levels," White said.

"Will he do that?" I asked dubiously.

"He'll do it." White was sure. As we continued to talk about Aaron, he observed, "You're very concerned."

We stared at him. Of course, we were concerned.

"I'm going to tell him that. Aaron thinks you don't care."

He called Aaron in and talked a bit about what we had said. Again I told Aaron he was psychotic and needed to take medication.

Aaron turned to White. "My parents think I'm psychotic. What do you think?"

"I think you're at risk," he said, frustrating me. We knew Aaron was very ill, way past at risk. As I saw it, he needed badly to hear the truth. Why else would he take medication? (Later I understood that a psychiatrist needs to protect his connection with his patient by avoiding a head-on confrontation. Aaron would have felt we were all united against him if White had agreed with me. But at the time it made me doubt White more.)

"I think you should try to stick it out at MIT," Arthur said. "Finish the work for your quantum course. Then you can leave in good standing and return when you're ready."

"I don't know if that's possible," Aaron said.

Arthur and I took our turn waiting while Aaron talked with White, who seemed pleased when he came out to say good-bye to us.

"That helped," he said. "It cleared the air."

Outside it was drizzling. As we walked to Arthur's car on a sidewalk bordered by fruit trees, we trod on little red balls.

"They're apples," I said. "Crabapples."

"No, they aren't. They're berries," Aaron said. But he tested my assertion by reaching up and pulling a little reddish fruit from a branch overhead, then squashing it his fingers.

"You're right," he said, seeing the core and seeds. "They're apples."

Perhaps this exchange stays in my mind because it was so ordinary, an unremarkable conversation about an unimportant point, in which evidence convinced Aaron, the kind of talk we could rarely have now that we lived in the land of insanity.

Aaron didn't want to go out with us to eat, so we drove back to Beacon Hill and let him off at his corner.

"I love you, Aaron," I said as he got out of the van.

We watched him cross the wet street and walk away, hunched against the rain.

For a few days I was encouraged by White's sense that our meeting had been helpful and Aaron would resume treatment. Then White called.

"I need to tell you that Aaron has decided to stop seeing me. I won't be taking care of him," he said.

"Things seem very bleak," I said.

"It's going to get worse before it gets better."

White had referred Aaron to another psychiatrist, who called a few days later. After one session Aaron had decided not to work with her.

"Our conversation was very preliminary," she said. "He was clearly delusional. He was talking about the way I used words like *the* and *and*."

"I see."

"He needs to be in a relationship with someone," she said.

That was a useless observation, I thought. It was too clear by now that what we thought Aaron needed and what he was willing to do did not coincide. Delusional, hostile, and frightened, he was altogether on his own. Despite Jay, despite friends, despite my therapist, despite Arthur's cooperation, I too felt alone with my burden of loss and sorrow, a feeling I had carried with me all my life.

Chapter 10

Arthur and I had set aside the idea of selling 311 East 9th Street. He wanted to move into Lanie's apartment on West 85th Street and I wanted to move back to 311. At least for the time being, I wanted the continuity the house provided with Aaron's past and my own, though it meant I would be dealing with repairs and upkeep, with state and city regulations, with finding a tenant for the occasional vacancy, and for figuring out how to pay the bills. In three years our mortgage from the Ukrainian credit union would end with a substantial balance due. By then I would have to decide whether to refinance or sell the house.

Starting in January I would be working at Seward Park High School, where my student teaching had led to a job for spring semester, a proper paying job with health benefits. Let me say that again: I had a real job, not just a few hours a week. And a real salary at last.

Before I moved back to 311, I had the apartment painted. Not wanting to sleep in the bedroom Arthur and I had shared, I set up my futon in the living room, a room that by itself was larger than my studio in Brooklyn; it felt luxurious to spread myself out in so much space. Living in my own house felt secure. I enjoyed our lively neighborhood: the coffee shops and restaurants I knew

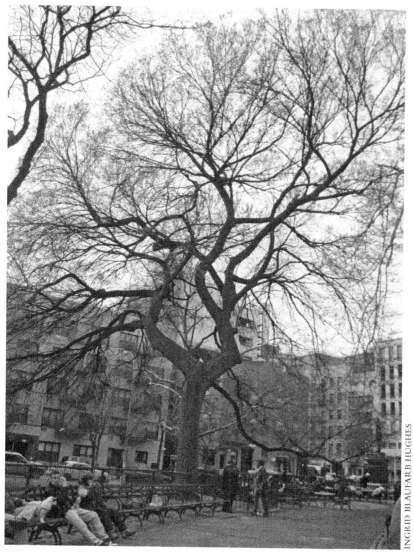

One of the great elms in Tompkins Square, New York City

well; the movie theaters and way-off Broadway shows. Tompkins Square had recently been renovated, with the possibly intended result of clearing the Hooverville where homeless people had lived, though a few had come back to sleep on the benches. Children shrieked cheerfully in the renovated playgrounds, and there were new plantings of shrubbery. Best of all, I loved the many great elms whose branches soared wide and high, crooking their elbows in patterns that shifted with my vantage point as I wandered through the park to the Tompkins Square Library.

My walk through the Lower East Side to work took me down First Avenue to Houston, then along Orchard and across Delancey—where nothing much was fancy except Ratner's, the wonderful dairy restaurant—and down Ludlow to the huge fortress of the high school.

My favorite class was a double period of a senior English class for immigrants, mostly from China, who needed help with their English. They were bright and full of questions; even those who neglected their work were respectful. I enjoyed them, as I had taken pleasure in Stasha and Aaron when they were in their teens. Together we read Anzia Yezierska's novel *Bread Givers*, set on the Lower East Side streets my students and I walked every day. The book concerns a family of Polish Jews, five daughters and their extraordinarily male chauvinist father. My students, often from strongly patriarchal families, easily recognized the conflicts between the father and his daughters. As they bent over their desks to write an in-class assignment, quiet would descend on the room, the creative quiet of twenty-eight students thinking out what they wanted to say, while I sat breathing in the peace.

That class was a pleasure. But I had three other classes and little idea how to structure a semester of instruction. Jay was full of clever suggestions for classroom activities, but I couldn't always make his ideas work. In the classroom I was aware of my lack of experience. Knowing that my sense of inadequacy was magnified by the helplessness I felt about Aaron didn't help me.

Besides teaching, I had to deal with report cards, parent-teacher evenings, observations by my supervisor. Later in the spring, when I was more comfortable in the classroom, I still felt beleaguered by the needs of a hundred students and unhappy that I had so little time for myself. What felt good was being part of a public high school, one of the most central American institutions, for the first time in my life. No longer was I on the periphery. I liked the feeling of the quiet school around me once the tide of students had drained from the building at two fifteen. Then I could take the stacks of student work I had collected during the day and zip them into my backpack, reviewing my classes mentally as I prepared to make my way home. And how satisfying it was to have a biweekly paycheck in a respectable amount. The small amounts I earned as a tutor at the Baruch Reading and Writing Lab had not been a living wage.

When the phone rang in the evenings, it was usually Aaron, raving again, calling daily to accuse me with great fury of acts that he would never name. The strain of preparing for the second of three comprehensive exams MIT required for a doctorate was aggravating his paranoia. "You have to stop it, Ingrid. You can't do these things. It's not legal."

"Do what?" I would say, perhaps staring out the tall window into the pitch-black void of the courtyard behind the house. Aaron always answered in the same baffling way.

"You *know*. You and Arthur are complicit. It's criminal, what you're doing."

"What is it you think we're doing?"

"Don't pretend you don't know. I know I'm being drugged. If ever I get the upper hand—things will be different."

"Aaron, you're being crazy."

"I'm not simply mad. If there was any way, *any* way, I would exercise it to seek reparations for the things being done to me. But I'm powerless. It's like I'm in a police state." It was wrenching to hear his words, and his threats were worrying.

"You could choose to take medication," I said. "You're not being drugged."

"I'm not sure you realize there are no choices."

Trapped in the circularity of Aaron's accusations and my questions, I was utterly frustrated—by his refusal to explain, by his rejection of medication, and by the impossibility of satisfying him. The steady pounding of his paranoia came to represent the hold his illness had over us all, the element of truth in his statement that there were no choices. If he had to live with his predicament, we had to also.

Despite his condition, he passed his exams, a testimony to his intelligence and stamina. "If you had been through what I've been through, you would curl up in fetal position for the rest of your life," he told me once. Maybe he was right. I tried to console myself with my knowledge of his strength. But this very strength, the independence he had shown since childhood, made it less likely that he would accept help.

Stasha had retreated to 311 a few months before my return, when the studio overlooking the garden on the second floor became vacant. She was working now at the Center for Cuban Studies and volunteering at the leftist radio station, WBAI, as well, "collecting sound," as she called it, for the evening news.

She was so often petulant and accusing that I suggested she and I have a session with Ellen Wachtel.

"How are you?" Ellen asked her. She looked to me both shaky and sad. Though she was a bit heavier than she had been—as I was—her face remained lovely.

"Things are pretty hard." She turned to me. "Do you realize how much has happened to me since you decided to leave Daddy?" she asked. "That was a big deal for me. Of course I'm angry at you. And Aaron's illness is big too."

"That's a tragedy for your family," Ellen said.

I was grateful for her acknowledgment of what we all felt. So many people tried to reassure me that Aaron would get better when they had no basis for such a prediction.

"Aaron's illness changes everything," I said. "Everything."

"I feel like it's contagious," Stasha said. "I want to help Aaron but it makes me so anxious."

At Ellen's suggestion, Arthur and I met with a psychiatrist it turned out neither of us liked, then tried another. The second one spoke of the benefits of a short hospitalization. It would allow Aaron to meet other psychiatric patients and maybe recognize that their suffering was similar to his. He would be supervised in taking his medication as well, perhaps getting him over the hump of his resistance. Arthur wouldn't hear of hospitalization. I was willing to try anything, but I couldn't see how we would get Aaron to agree. We had no legal grounds to have him hospitalized against his will. He had said nothing to make us think he might hurt himself or anyone else.

After a few sessions, I decided this doctor wasn't quite right. This time Ellen suggested Chris Beels. "He's good; you'll like him." She offered to call and ask him to take us on.

"Why do we need to see another psychiatrist?" Arthur asked me when I reported that Ellen had reached Dr. Beels and he would work with us.

"Don't you want to do the best we can for Aaron?" I said. So Arthur agreed.

Chris Beels turned out to be a man in his sixties, upright, relaxed, kindly. He reminded me of the faculty at the boarding school Arthur and I had attended in Colorado, outdoorsmen at ease on the ski slopes or in the classroom. He gave us steaming mugs of herbal tea before he listened to me tell our story yet again. He was gifted at picking out the positives of the situation, and for the first time I had confidence in a psychiatrist and as a result some lightening of my mood. Arthur too liked him.

I wrote a letter along lines Chris proposed, suggesting Aaron apply for a medical leave from MIT as a way to give him more options. If he found a therapist who would take his knowledge and experience seriously, someone he could negotiate with, he would be more able to stay out of the hospital. Arthur sent a similar letter. Neither succeeded.

At Chris's suggestion, we made yet another trip to Boston. In the middle of a March blizzard, we made our way to Aaron's to take him out to supper. Despite deep snow and rain coming on top of it, he wore a lightweight leather jacket over a sweater, jeans, and his leather lace-ups because he had no boots. This inability to clothe himself properly was another sign of illness, since he had always dressed sensibly. But Aaron hadn't given up: his shoes were shined, an attempt to waterproof them.

Over dinner at a little restaurant near his apartment, we laid out the different possibilities we had discussed with Chris Beels. Aaron could try to stay at MIT, he could try to get a medical leave, he could simply withdraw. We wanted him to agree to treatment. But it was no surprise that he wouldn't. He talked angrily, tightening his lips against his teeth and spitting out his words. As soon as we finished eating, he sent us away. I crawled into bed at the John Jeffries House, the quiet hotel where I was staying, and fell into a deep sleep of depression and exhaustion.

In fact, Aaron had already decided to withdraw from MIT, as I learned from his letter to the head of the physics department, which was turned over to us after his death.

> This letter confirms what we spoke about in your office this past Wednesday, that for personal reasons I am withdrawing from graduate study at MIT.

> Elizabeth Bishop wrote that the sea
> is like what we imagine knowledge to be
> dark, salt, clear, moving, utterly free,
> drawn from the cold hard mouth
> of the world, derived from the rocky breasts
> forever, flowing and drawn, and since
> our knowledge is historical, flowing and flown.

> I only add that the sensation of knowing and the process of discovery waver in their proximity.

Reading Aaron's letter for the umpteenth time, I find myself wondering what was in his mind when he quoted Elizabeth Bishop's poem. His words sound perfectly sane, if cryptic. Was he thinking of the cruelty of "the cold hard mouth of the world"? or the loss of his understanding, which had seemed "flowing," and was now "flown"? Could he have recognized his difficulties as a loss of understanding? Or was he thinking about the nature of knowledge in some other way? I wonder especially what he meant by his final sentence about the relationship of discovery to the "sensation of knowing."

Perhaps Aaron felt some relief once he had officially withdrawn from MIT. Chatting with him a few days later, I reported that I could see one solitary daffodil blooming in the garden from my desk.

"That makes it all the more special," he said with his old kindness. And months past his twenty-fifth birthday, he agreed I could send him a gift. He needed a cooking pot; he had burned one. I chose a kettle and a saucepan at Macy's and had them sent to Boston, pleased there was something I could give him, no matter how basic.

When Aaron had to leave graduate school, he lost the chance to pursue his studies in physics and the prestige of being at MIT. Though it was far from the most serious of my troubles, I too had lost the status, vicarious but real, of having a child in a doctoral program at a famous university. Now I was someone else, the mother of a son with schizophrenia. I soon learned to be wary of bringing this up. Some friends were frightened. Most were clueless. "Was it your fault?" one woman asked. Others gave advice. Aaron shouldn't be alone in his condition, one told me—as if he would let me near him. One suggested he visit her farm because it would be good therapy to work outdoors growing things. Someone else thought he might form a relationship with a woman that would change him. Usually, I was able to disregard these responses, which I knew reflected the attitudes that pervaded our world, which had been mine as well. But they left me feeling more alone with Aaron's illness.

Chris Beels had more ideas, which involved writing to Aaron once again with new proposals, though what they were I no longer remember. Beels himself wrote to Aaron as well.

Aaron responded in May:

Dear Ingrid:

I'm reluctant to respond to your most recent letter only because any response might encourage you to write more. However, it is threatening to become an ongoing joke if you continue sending these things. Very considerate you are indeed, and well meaning is your Dr. Beels. However, I would appreciate it most sincerely if you would put to rest your imploring attempts to have me seek psychiatric help. . . . One thing that I can say for sure is that telling me I'm insane is not going to bring us any closer. . . .

Your not so-loving son,

Aaron

At Chris Beels's suggestion, I began at last to educate myself. From memoirs like Mark Vonnegut's *Eden Express* and compilations of accounts by schizophrenics, I got an idea—I'm afraid a rather limited idea—of what mental illness felt like. I found a good introduction to the issues of schizophrenia in E. Fuller Torrey's *Surviving Schizophrenia: A Manual for Families, Patients, and Providers,* which describes the illness and how it damages the structures and systems of the brain. In ways we don't yet understand, this damage caused Aaron to hallucinate voices insulting him, as well as smells, like the body odor that so disturbed him at Swarthmore, and the noxious air he complained of later, and strange tastes, which made food or drink taste bad, supporting his belief that he was being poisoned. Because for the most part he kept his experience to himself, all we can know with certainty is that he lived in a world that wasn't ours, but far more menacing. The abuse he perceived hurt and frightened him, as it would anyone. Arthur's and my cooperation in persecuting him, as he imagined, was a further cruelty. No wonder he felt powerless. No wonder he was angry at us.

Torrey's book has striking images showing the differences in structure between the brains of identical twins, one with schizophrenia and one without it. Loss of brain tissue has been found in many different studies, both those that compare brain scans of those living with schizophrenia to those of a twin, and by postmortem studies. But we know there are people with schizophrenia who do demanding intellectual work, so evidently it's possible to function with some of these losses.

In addition, the brains of people with schizophrenia have neurochemical changes involving several neurotransmitters, of which dopamine, serotonin, and glutamate have been among the most studied. There are also electrical, immunological, and inflammatory abnormalities. The various parts of the brain affected include the limbic system, the amygdala, the hippocampus, and the hypothalamus.

After reading about these changes, I understood better that Aaron's illness was biologically based, and not a result of his experience. This was an important inroad into my ignorance.

As I write in early 2016, the big news in the biology of schizophrenia is a research finding based on a study of nearly 65,000 people by scientists at the Broad Institute and Harvard Medical School. For the first time, researchers have identified a specific gene, C4, and have good evidence for their theory of how it produces symptoms of schizophrenia. C4 can have up to four copies of varying forms in different individuals. This gene controls pruning of synapses, or neural connections, a normal development in the adolescent brain. It seems that some variations of C4 produce excessive pruning, causing symptoms of schizophrenia. Most likely, in the next few years research will reveal other genes that play a role in schizophrenia and more knowledge about how they function.

Doctors describe the causes of schizophrenia in terms of risk factors, the strongest of which is having relatives with mental illness. In other words, a person's genetic makeup can increase the risk of schizophrenia. Generally genes are thought to create a predisposition which environmental factors interact with. Arthur's mother talked freely of a breakdown following Arthur's birth, which he believes was a psychotic depression. She told us stories of voices or presences that appeared when she was distressed. In our ignorance, Arthur and I considered these to be manifestations of her California flakiness, along with her interest in séances and her special powers. Now I have more respect for her ability to keep going, living by herself or with a boarder at her big house in Ojai, California, visiting Naushon or traveling abroad. In my family my father's sister had suffered a breakdown, though nobody talked about this. I knew her to be sensible, cheerful, generous, and happy in her marriage and her career as a painter and sculptor.

Environmental risk factors include a winter or spring birth, perhaps because pregnant women are more likely to contract a virus in winter, changing the fetal environment and contributing to the later development of schizophrenia. Aaron was born in January, and I had had a cold during my pregnancy with him. Problems at birth are another factor. Aaron's delivery was induced by my obstetrician as a matter of his convenience. Population statistics also show that people raised in cities are more likely to have schizophrenia. But many millions of people have relatives with mental illnesses, a winter birth, an urban upbringing, and even an induced birth, and still grow up free of schizophrenia, so none of these factors by itself, nor even in combination with all the others, is decisive.

Chris Beels suggested a support group that met at St. Vincent's Hospital, just a walk across town from our house. I attended a number of times and listened as each woman talked about her son or daughter in hospital or in a halfway house. But these mothers were dealing with a different set of problems from ours. Their children lived often in supportive housing and seemed to communicate with them willingly. They understood they were sick and took medication. I had begun to see, though intermittently, that Aaron was going to live on his own with his illness.

This recognition was encouraged by Chris, who suggested, not for the first time, that we find a way to live with Aaron's condition.

"What do you mean?" I asked.

"I think you could try to open up negotiations with him about work, about some kind of visiting arrangement. Get all the possibilities out and help him consider them." But I wasn't able to do that.

Sometimes when we talked Aaron was angry. "Boston is a disgusting city," he might say. Or he might be reading Elizabeth Bishop and comment on her poetry. Other times he wouldn't answer his phone. He told Arthur that he was entertaining himself by watching videos, seeing "how little I can do for the greatest amount of time." Chris Beels thought he was in a catatonic state, a condition of disorganization and lack of will.

Aaron asked my opinion of him one day and listened to it. He agreed he was the age for mental illness to strike. But no, he was sure that wasn't the problem, and he was very amusing in his repudiation of it. His moments of near-lucidity teased me, encouraging me to feel he might after all accept the need to treat his illness.

I think now that Aaron's consideration of whether he might be mentally ill was a product of his strong intellect. He couldn't avoid knowing that it was one explanation of his experience. But it made no sense to him.

When I reeducated myself in order to write this book, I learned what kept Aaron from awareness of his own illness. Unlike the psychological defense we call denial, Aaron's problem is called anosognosia and results from damage to the brain. It has been recognized in those with brain damage for many years, for instance in the stroke victim who insists he can control a paralyzed leg. Only since the 1990s has it been studied as an issue for people with schizophrenia.

Most of us are well aware of alterations in our mental abilities: we notice when we're intoxicated or forgetful or dulled by fatigue. It's hard for us to imagine that we might experience major changes in sensory perception, much less hallucinations, and fail to register that something is amiss. Aaron's illness blocked him from recognizing his illness. And I failed to understand his experience, and so failed to understand how much I didn't understand.

As the large balance due on our mortgage on 311 East 9th Street loomed, I fretted over what to do. Refinancing at the credit union on Second Avenue turned out to be impossible; they were no longer offering mortgages for commercial property, as our house was designated because of our six apartments. Other banks considered us either too small or too big.

I showed the house to realtors to get an idea of its value, and to several couples considering sharing ownership with me. Telling people about the history of our old house made me feel rather grand. But these showings were a strain; I felt the house I owned and lived in as a part of me, a protective carapace that I had to present for evaluation. Before each showing I had to ask the tenants to clear the halls of odds and ends that collected by their doors. I dashed around to put our apartment in order. The boiler in the low, dark cellar was usually my starting point, where a tall visitor had to bend to avoid banging his head on the pipes. We walked up through our apartment, spent a few minutes in the garden, glanced at a couple of tenant apartments on the upper floors, and finally climbed to the roof overlooking 9th Street. This went on for months, without producing an offer I wanted to accept.

That summer Jay and I were in Hebron, New York, a tiny hamlet an hour east of Saratoga Springs. After not writing for a year, I found myself facing a blank page. The one story I began wouldn't jell. Nor did the poems I attempted, usually descriptions of what was around me. Now that I didn't have teaching to distract me I couldn't avoid my sense of desolation. Aaron was languishing in Boston, refusing to let us near him. I hadn't seen him since the snowy, icy March night when Arthur and I took him out to dinner.

"I can't write," I told Jay as we sat on the little balcony of the rather odd house where we were staying, overlooking a lawn surrounded by woods.

"How can you change that?" he asked. "What do you need to do to be able to write?"

"There's nothing I can do," I said. I had stopped thinking it possible. I tried to guide myself through my days with the least damage, as I told myself, trying to let Jay function, trying not to wail all the time. During sex I broke into sobs and couldn't continue. "I make myself inconsolable," I noted. "If I can't have Aaron, I'd rather feel my loss. Loss is real. Being happy is frightening." I had always had a tendency to consider happiness less reliable than sorrow. Now I felt that it would separate me from Aaron.

It didn't help that Jay and I seemed to be lost in the middle of nowhere. Evenings we would often drive the local roads that wandered among the fields of corn or grass, connecting to other roads through more fields and past occasional houses and barns. One night we took a new road that led to the top of a ridge with a view, an exciting change; it was so rare to get a perspective. Returning to our house, we passed a dead end sign and kept going till we stopped the car on the circular turnaround. The hills and trees rose up around us to close us in.

Stasha had quit her job at the Center for Cuban Studies and stopped helping with the evening news at WBAI. Instead she was word processing and answering phones as a temporary worker uptown, while complaining that she was bored and had to dress up for work. On the phone she was disgruntled and critical of me.

When I protested, she said, "Well, I do harbor anger at you. But it's not permanent."

"But you're angry at me during most of our conversations."

"I would like to talk to you. But you don't know how to do anything but give advice."

"Right. I shouldn't advise you. I have to say it's hard not to when you complain so much. But I'll work on it."

"And you treat me with kid gloves. It makes me uneasy. You don't have the attitude that I'm OK."

While I never at any time doubted that Stasha was OK, which in our family now meant not suffering from a major mental illness, she was plainly unhappy. I couldn't see why she had quit a meaningful job to do temp work.

"She thinks she's supporting me when in fact she's impatient and talks down to me," I told Jay. "At the same time, she wants me to take care of her. And I feel she should be taking care of me!" I threw up my hands with exasperation at myself, at her, at our predicament. Jay laughed.

In August I took a bus across Massachusetts to meet Arthur and Stasha in Boston, although Aaron had made it clear he didn't want to see us. Ringing his bell got no response. Neither did standing in the narrow street and calling his name. I was sure he was home, as he later confirmed. After lunch we tried again, pressing his bell over and over, yelling "Aaron, Aaarooon." We failed again. So we went on to meet with a therapist Chris Beels had recommended. When we had told our story, he commented that Arthur's and my separation could not have caused Aaron's illness, although it could have supplied him with delusional material. This made me feel a little better for a time. He suggested that we not let ourselves be controlled by Aaron's illness. Excellent advice, which I recorded in my journal. Perhaps I should say I entombed it in my journal.

On our return to the city, I looked for part-time work. Teaching public school in the spring semester had enabled me to pay down my debts, but it had been draining. In October I began teaching a night course twice a week at La Guardia Community College in Queens. After the winter holidays, I would be at Baruch, a short walk away from home—the woman who supervised the reading courses there liked me.

In New York I felt more secure, in the city throbbing, sometimes shrieking with life, from the structures below our feet, the trains and water mains and utility lines, to the streets congested with people, bikes, buses, taxis, delivery trucks, and wailing fire engines, to the buildings rising into the air, with their layers of apartments and offices. Braced by the avenues and streets of the urban grid, in touch with my friends, able to see Stasha rather than listen to her complaints on the phone, I seemed able to think better. It came to me that I could write a memoir about my relationship with my father, focusing on our years in Saigon in the fifties and our battles over political questions.

Jay had planned to spend a month in the fall cat-sitting for a neighbor while he looked for a place for the academic year. He stayed with me at 311 until our friend left for a month in Europe. But as he was installing himself in her apartment, I was prickly.

"Are you upset that I'm not with you?" He was standing by the door on his way out as he spoke, frowning slightly.

"I guess I am. It's hard to be alone now." Though I felt I was giving up my vaunted independence, I wanted Jay's company. So Stasha agreeably took over cat-sitting, and Jay officially moved in. He had Stasha's old room on the garden level to write in and do his class preparation. And without much deliberation, we were living together.

Stasha I were cooking together when I opened a jar of what I thought were my mother's preserves, put up several years earlier.

It turned out to be a little plum pudding, a welcome treat. While Stasha cooked I read *British Cookery*, a volume of traditional recipes that my father hadn't been able to give up from my mother's collection of cookbooks.

"What's wrong, Mom? You've got your forlorn look," Stasha asked briskly. I liked her astringent response.

"It makes me sad, reading Granma's book."

"You should cry more. You wouldn't be so anxious if you cried," she said firmly. She was probably right. But I wasn't good at crying.

In December Arthur visited Aaron, finding him painfully thin, with shadows under his eyes and a strained expression, working a lot on his computer. There was no food in the house. I worried that Aaron would starve himself.

The truth was worse, as Katherine told us after his death. Earlier that month he had tried to take his life by forging a prescription for codeine and taking it all. But it hadn't worked. He hadn't been able to keep it down.

What must he have gone through to reach the point of downing a bottle of codeine? What despair must he have felt? What anger at the way he was bedeviled by a hostile world, by our cooperation with those who wanted to hurt him, to control him? For how long had he been considering this act, while reporting to us that he was lying around and watching dollar videos? What resolution did it take, what planning, to forge a prescription, get hold of the codeine, and drink it down?

I am so grateful he didn't die then, grateful we were spared finding his decayed body in his Boston apartment, grateful for the time that lay ahead when he was home again.

Chapter 11

My father often mentioned his visits to Dossie Friar during our telephone talks. When he announced he had a friend, I knew it could only be Dossie. It would be a lie if I said I was happy for my father. Instead, despite all my mixed feelings about him, I feared another loss. Now he would probably revert to his old attitude of inattention, punctuated a couple of times a year by visits.

This year, knowing he was unlikely to receive another invitation for Christmas, I asked him to join me and Jay and Stasha in New York. When my mother was alive, Christmas had been a great gathering at the farm. Nora's and David's and my families would occupy every bed and cot and the couches in the living room. The air would be thick with the history that connected us, so dense it felt to me as buoyant as water, even as it sloughed away much of the person I was in New York, and rendered me daughter, sister, mother, wife, as my parents saw me.

Now my father, Stasha, Jay, and I were a remnant of the family. Aaron maintained his isolation in Boston. My brother Billy had been far away for so long I had grown accustomed to not seeing him. But I missed my Washington brother and sister and their families, and I knew my father would miss them as well. Without my siblings and their children to buffer my father's criticisms, it would be harder to get through a week with him. He didn't like New York, he didn't like the way I kept house, and he always let me know his feelings. I began to dread his visit.

"I'm trying to decide how to handle Granpa when he starts complaining," I told Stasha. She was living with us until January, when she was going to transplant herself to San Francisco.

"Just let out an earsplitting scream," she said.

My father had grown an Abraham Lincoln beard at Dossie's suggestion. She thought it made him look more handsome, while I thought, when he arrived for his visit, that it obscured his face. I gave him a hug, hung up his coat, and sat him down for tea and cake.

"I want to get married," he said. "But Dossie hasn't said yes. She doesn't think her children, or mine, will be pleased if we get married."

"It's fine with me if you get married," I lied politely.

"She's concerned about her own children and grandchildren," he said. "And then there's my health." Considering my father's regular bouts of bronchial pneumonia and periodic hospital emergencies, I could see why Dossie would fear another bereavement before many years passed.

"But I can't live like this," he said. "I can't get used to being alone. Anyway, Dossie doesn't want me to tell people about our relationship."

"OK."

"He told his sister too," I told Jay later, with no compunction, after I had talked with my aunt on the phone. I felt a good deal of bitterness that this man who had withheld from me the truth of his work was now so ready to disclose the secret Dossie wanted him to keep, though the silence she sought was no more than a fig leaf. Her children, who visited her farm often, knew my father was usually there better than I did. But it was a fig leaf she wanted to keep in place.

"What do you hear from Aaron?" my father asked. I mentioned Arthur's visit, his report that Aaron didn't look well.

"Surely, you can have him committed to a hospital."

"No. We can't. He's twenty-five years old."

"But he can't take care of himself."

"That's the way the law is."

"There must be a way."

"Not unless he's willing. Unless he's a danger to himself or others, he can't be held against his will." I was annoyed. Why would you expect anything to be done right in a society which cared so poorly for the frail and needy? Why could my father not recognize that?

As I had anticipated, he complained a lot. I needed a new coffee maker; I should have better lighting in the dining room. I should buy a new pocketbook. Why did people live in New York, when it was full of bad air and trash? After a couple of days, I made a protest.

"You know, Daddy, I look forward to your coming so much," I lied again. "And then you complain all the time. You don't want me to feel you're picking on me."

"I'm a cranky old man. That's the New York tradition—bickering." He meant his mother had bickered with her children a lot.

"Well, it's a tradition we should stop."

"I'll try." And then he was better.

"The diplomat's daughter," I congratulated myself, a little sarcastically.

Stasha had shot footage for a short video about Ecuadorian street vendors who sold clothing and textiles on Canal Street, and a friend had helped her edit it. She was applying to graduate programs in film; the video she was making would be part of her application. In January she flew to San Francisco and set herself up, calling friends of friends to establish connections, spending time with her college buddy Samirah Alkasim, finding an apartment, finding a therapist. She decided against film school, but got part-time work helping a woman make a documentary film.

After Stasha told me Aaron had been talking about AIDS orphans, I called and reminded him that he wasn't an orphan. I was his mother. Arthur was his father.

"I've seen this movie before," he said angrily.

"Some movies you have to see a lot of times." He calmed down, and we talked for a long time. I had slept poorly, worrying about issues related to the house, and in my fatigue something made me begin to cry.

"Poor Ingrid. You really are a wreck," Aaron said kindly.

But often he wouldn't talk to us, or even deposit checks we sent him. After he complained to Arthur that he hadn't received money J.M. Forbes was supposed to send for from Arthur's mother, Arthur made a call and the problem was corrected. But Aaron accused him of interfering. He should tell J.M. Forbes not to send him money. He didn't need it. Arthur ignored this demand, but Aaron continued to reject help from me, Arthur, and Arthur's mother, though not consistently.

———

On my father's seventy-sixth birthday, Dossie agreed to marry him. His news left me too dismayed to speak. Why? Why, when I found him so irritating, did I feel apprehensive about his marriage, especially since it would relieve me of the burden of traveling to West Virginia every time he was sick?

"Aren't you going to congratulate me?" he asked.

"That's great. Congratulations." I spoke mechanically.

"Sound happy," he demanded. "Show some enthusiasm."

"I'm very happy for you. That's wonderful." I could lie, but enthusiasm was more than I could muster.

Not that I had anything against Dossie, but I expected I would soon. Anybody who would choose to be close to my father must share his attitudes and be uncongenial to me. Now he would live at Dossie's farm, buried even deeper in West Virginia than my parents had been, and be taken over by her family of three sons, each with a wife and two daughters, who came up often in his conversation.

As I continued to worry about 311, it came to me that if Jay and I moved to the fourth floor, a smaller, more suitable apartment, and rented out the garden duplex, I could cover our expenses. I started the work of bringing the house up to code in order to qualify for a new mortgage. The halls were plastered and painted, the joist of the staircase was reinforced. The house morphed from a protective carapace to a complicated burden I couldn't put down. But I couldn't give it up.

At Baruch I taught my two reading courses diligently but without excitement, guiding students to dig into the immigrant stories we read, preparing them at semester end for their reading test. On weekends I would meet a friend at a café, or if the weather was good, we would sit in Tompkins Square. Leaving the park, I would often stop at the library to search the shelves for a novel or a memoir. Jay and I would eat out at the Tibetan place or Casa Linga or an Indian restaurant. We might go to a movie in the neighborhood. But more and more I limited myself to my familiar rounds. The space Aaron had made for Ingridity was narrower now.

To Jay I complained that I was fed up with metaphor, sick of the meanings that poets found oozing from ordinary objects. Particularly oozy was Galway Kinnell's poem, "Blackberry Eating," posted in many subway cars. In the poem the berries become words, and eating them a metaphor for making poems. Poets make the most of the human capacity to see meaning, which is distorted in people with schizophrenia. Aaron saw everything as swollen, bulging with meaning, often a threatening meaning, the way people do in altered states of consciousness. In my misery I saw the truth as lacking meaning. My berries were berries. That was it. Plain old berries.

I suppose it was my deepening depression that made teaching in a summer program at Baruch more appealing than going away that year. The previous summer's unhappiness in rural New York was not anything to repeat. Because class met four mornings a week and I spent the afternoons reading student work and preparing for the next day, I was soon immersed. My students were engaged as well, rewarding me for my hard work.

As the summer wore on, Aaron grew increasingly remote, though he did let us know he was planning to leave his apartment despite being in no position to get another. Arthur and I talked with Chris Beels, who thought Aaron was trying to manage without us and might become homeless.

"What can we do?" I asked Chris.

"If you intervene, he may pull away more," he said.

Chris was usually so optimistic that I was shaken by his assessment. At lunch after our session, Arthur talked of his fear that Aaron would be on the streets and unable to protect himself. An image of Aaron suffering injury to his brain bothered him, the brain schizophrenia had already injured.

The end of August was fast approaching, the date when Aaron would be without a roof over his head. Trudging up Second Avenue to Baruch to make copies of my fall syllabus, I found myself in a rage of anxiety so acute I could hardly bear it, with a feeling of meaninglessness and sorrow, a sense of having done wrong, not in any specific way, but in a deeper, more general one, the sort of feeling you might have in a dream.

At last Aaron told Arthur he "could use some help" moving out of his apartment. With my fall classes starting before Labor Day, I had to leave this to Arthur and Stasha. Stasha thought out an approach with her California therapist and flew home. She and I and Arthur met with Chris Beels, so she would be well prepared when she got to Boston.

There she found Aaron flat on his back on the bare floor, having sold his mattress with most of his other furniture. He was rather sick because, as he put it, "I volunteered for medical research." I was aghast at Stasha's report. Medical research that left him sick? What could that be?

Through the next days Arthur, Stasha, and Aaron reported to me often. It turned out that Aaron had concluded on his own that he was schizophrenic. Seeking help with housing, he had talked to an outreach worker from the Freedom Trail Clinic at the Lindemann Mental Health Center not far from his apartment. There he met with a psychiatrist who confirmed his

self-diagnosis. At this doctor's request, he had agreed to participate in a study that required a spinal tap, causing him such headaches that now he couldn't get up.

The psychiatrist he saw, Dr. Goff, noted that Aaron dated his
social withdrawal from the fall of 1987, as he had when he saw
Dr. White. As we learned from Goff's notes after Aaron's death:

> [Aaron] felt he was repulsive, worthless. Describes embarrass-
> ing self by "inappropriate" lecture at college. Fall 91 devel-
> oped ideas of reference, meaning to colors, paranoia, drop in
> concentration. Doesn't believe he was depressed. Was not
> using drugs. Believed he was being "graded" by news an-
> chors on TV. Has doubts about whether he really exists. At-
> tempted OD by codeine Dec 93. Vomited it up. Believes he
> can sweat out fluid instead of urinating. Family is not aware
> of patient's problems. Patient acknowledges hypochondriacal
> family. "Lies around" has difficulty w hygiene & eating.

Aaron's doubt about his own existence is a not uncommon
symptom of schizophrenia, which psychiatrists describe as an
altered sense of self. Goff's impression of Aaron was that he was

> well-groomed, . . . very articulate, converses spontaneously,
> affect appropriate, organized. ideas of reference, hears people
> say what he is thinking. Believes he puts words in other peo-
> ple's mouths. Aural hallucinations, olfactory & gustatory hal-
> lucinations. Acrid odor. No amnesia, visual illusions.

At the Freedom Trail Clinic, Stasha and Arthur met Dr. Goff,
who felt Aaron would soon agree to treatment—medication and
therapy. His condition on medication was predicted by his level

of functioning before his breakdown, he told Arthur and Stasha. (Chris Beels also felt Aaron's high level of adjustment before his illness was the most encouraging factor in his history.)

What a breakthrough! Aaron understood that he was suffering from schizophrenia. I had thought this could never happen. Would everything change now? I allowed myself to imagine that he might recover enough to resume his studies or perhaps work. The thought that he might rejoin the family brought me to tears.

But on the phone Aaron greeted me with suspicion. "I'm fine," he said.

"You're fine? Stasha said you were sick."

"I'm not well physically. Spiritually I'm fine. Everyone else is much more worried than I am. What did Stasha tell you?"

"She said you were lying down and couldn't get up."

"Did you know she was planning to visit? Why did she decide to come?"

"She wanted to see you. You said you needed help moving."

"I just want to know what you were thinking. It would be helpful to know what everyone was thinking."

As Aaron persisted in his interrogation, I extricated myself from the conversation, not wanting to say something that would feed his paranoia. But I was discouraged. If Aaron was in this suspicious frame of mind, I doubted he would agree to treatment.

Arthur and Stasha helped Aaron move those belongings he wanted to keep to a self-storage building. They drove him to the residence that had been arranged for him by someone at the Lindemann Center. Passing several ill people outside, the three of them went in and looked around. Aaron didn't like what he saw. On the street again he took off with a small backpack of his basics, all he carried with him after that. According to Arthur, when Aaron parted with them, "he looked like a mad person, insisting that we not contact him."

I was distraught. Aaron was off on his own, who knew where. We had no way to reach him. On the other hand, I still believed that at some level he understood he was ill with schizophrenia, as he had told the people at the Freedom Trail Clinic.

On Stasha's return, the two of us headed out for a walk through Tompkins Square and across the avenues of the Lower East Side, where the tenement buildings were covered with beer ads and graffiti. In the East River Park, we followed the river down toward the Williamsburg Bridge. As a cyclist zipped by us, I asked Stasha if she thought Aaron would be able to ride his bike if he got better. His bike had been such a pleasure to him before he got sick.

"Dr. Goff said that if he took medication Aaron would be almost symptom-free."

The thought of Aaron on his bike, or able to walk with us in the park, made me cry again. What a gift that would be.

But Aaron remained unreachable. Though he called a few days later from a motel, he wouldn't say where it was. He returned to the Freedom Trail Clinic a few weeks later for an interview with a social worker, who helped him apply for disability benefits from Medicare. After that he received disability and Medicare coverage and so had access to health care independently of us. The social worker's notes record Aaron's description of himself as "completely psychotic" while he was at MIT, an understanding that was short-lived and perhaps partial at best. But once my hopes had been raised, it took time for me to abandon them.

———

My father and Dossie chose Columbus Day weekend for their wedding.

"I want you to make a toast," my father said. "You should speak for four minutes. You can mention that I was born at Brooklyn Jewish Hospital. And you can bring in amusing family quirks. That we were frequently late for planes, though we never actually missed one. Dossie's sons can respond in kind."

"Are you planning to write their speeches too? Should I say I'm giving an authorized toast?"

"No. No. No. You shouldn't." My father sounded horrified, and after that didn't try to dictate what I should say in the toast he had commanded.

The wedding and reception took place at the Cosmos Club in Washington, a bastion of privilege that had for much of its history excluded minorities and women from membership. Even as we gathered in the ornate reception rooms under monstrous chandeliers, I had no idea what I would say in my toast.

It was my job to help my seven young nieces and stepnieces, the daughters of my sister and brother and my new stepbrothers, rehearse a cheer the girls had come up with. I marched them off to a wide marble hall leading to a reading room furnished with elderly gentlemen sunk in leather armchairs. The girls stood in their flowered party dresses and shrieked out, "Dyna-mite! Dyna-mite! Dossie and Dougie are dyna-mite!" On the final yell they hurled themselves into the air, routing one of the elderly gents, who folded his newspaper as he marched off. Much to my satisfaction. Distinguished elite have enough privileges, I thought, especially if male. Power to the next generation of girls!

When the time came, I stood next to my father in his tweed jacket and Dossie in an elegant aqua dress, her white curls around her face. I opened my mouth and found myself saying I hadn't seen my father so happy for a long time and how pleased I was that he would join Dossie on her farm, which suited his tastes so well. I thought I had done my job, but my father didn't.

"Make a toast," my father said. "Make a toast!"

I had not accomplished the essential task. So I concluded by asking the guests to drink to my father and Dossie, who I hoped would live to be 120 and have dozens of great-grandchildren. Several people praised me for the evident sincerity of my pleasure in my father's marriage. Was I telling the truth? I've never known.

As Jay and I got home from Washington, we were greeted by neighbors sitting on our stoop in the mild October sun.

"Aaron was looking for you," said José, a Construction Brigade *compañero* of Aaron's.

"Aaron?" I was stunned.

"Aaron. Your son, Aaron." José was disturbed by my bewilderment.

"When was he here?"

"A while ago. Half an hour, maybe."

Indoors I was upset that I had missed Aaron, but so tired I could do no more than make myself a cup of tea and sit down with it. Before long the buzzer sounded. I opened the apartment door for Aaron, as he stood warily back for someone coming down the stairs. He watched till she had left the house, then turned to me and held out his hand. When I reached up to embrace him, he offered a pretend hug, his body stiff and unyielding.

I pulled myself together. "Sit down, Aaron. Would you like

a cup of tea? Or something to eat? Are you going to stay? We have a bed for you," I said.

"No thanks. I just came to deal with my stuff in the cellar." He went down to check on the tools he had bought during his time as a carpenter, looked around, and went off again, leaving me in despair.

He reappeared the next day. There was scaffolding on the front of the building and workers were pointing the brick. The architect had stopped by and was talking to the contractor. Paying no attention to the commotion, Aaron carried cartons of his schoolwork from the cellar out to the trashcans, where he deposited them intact. I followed him down to the cellar when he went down again.

We stood under the low ceiling, facing shelves holding boxes of books, his and Stasha's schoolwork, camping gear, all the miscellany of a family storage room. In the dim light of an overhead fixture, Aaron was searching through boxes.

"Why are you carrying around a French grammar? Are you going to Quebec?" I was remembering his Christmas travels several years earlier.

"Hit the road, Jack," he said cryptically, and headed up the stairs with another load. Once he had left, I was able to rescue his boxes of notebooks and schoolwork. They have proved invaluable in writing about him.

He disappeared. Again I despaired. Then Arthur got a call. Aaron was going to Paris. Without a real good-bye, he was gone.

Loss, absence, and more loss, and more absence—how can you define these negatives? They lay sometimes below consciousness. But when I saw a young man who resembled Aaron, I thought of him, of how he used to look. I knew well that his skin was now likely to be a grayish color, his face shifting from unhappy to frightened.

Several weeks went by before we got another phone call. Aaron was in Paris, he was working on his French, we could write him *poste restante*, or general delivery. I did, and received a sarcastic answer.

Dear Ingrid,

I received your card of the 11 November. Having a wonderful time. Hope this finds you in good health. Give my regards to the others.

At least it was an answer. We had a way to communicate.

Jay and I drove to Three Churches, West Virginia, for Dossie's big family Thanksgiving, my father's only relatives attending. I was nervous as we arrived on foreign ground and were greeted by a several welcoming Friars. Surrounded by the families of two of Dossie's sons, we sat down to eat. As Dossie fussed over the food, urging seconds and thirds on everyone, her children and grandchildren teased her. But it was clear that they respected her, and they took my father in stride. Still I found it a strain to be in this house full of strangers, which had swallowed my father up.

When Dossie noticed, with what I came to learn was her characteristic sensitivity, that I wasn't feeling well, I had to admit I had a fierce headache. I was grateful that she sent me off to lie down in the dark living room, while everyone else gathered in the sitting room for charades.

The creak of the door opening woke me from my nap. I switched on a lamp and saw Dossie's granddaughters slipping in.

"Aunt Ingrid, you're so pretty," said the first one, standing by the couch.

"What?" I said, not believing my ears.

"You're so pretty. Your hair is pretty." She stroked my hair, as the other little girls came in.

"Feel Aunt Ingrid's hair," said my first admirer to her cousins. "Isn't it soft?"

Now Dossie stood at the door. "There you are, girls. Are you tormenting Ingrid?"

"They aren't tormenting me," I said. "They're taking care of me." It was lovely having the childish hands caress me, the childish voices praise me. For three years I had been toughing out Aaron's raging hostility, the raw hurt of his absence, and more recently, Stasha's absence in San Francisco as well. Dossie could have no idea how hungry I was for such simple appreciation.

Chapter 12

In January of 1995 Jay and I moved to the fourth floor. I had already lined up tenants for the duplex; their deposit and first month's rent would pay off a good chunk of our real estate tax arrears. But there was still work to be done on the house before I could get a new mortgage.

Early in the new year, Arthur heard from Aaron in Paris. He was moving from one inexpensive hotel to another and looking for an apartment. His bankcard gave him access to his Boston account, supplied by contributions from me and Arthur and a small amount of Supplemental Security Income. "He sounded more or less together, laughing in his nervous way a couple of times. He said he doesn't like talking to anyone who knows English," Arthur told me. Asked about his visa, Aaron said that since his passport hadn't been stamped at the airport, there was no record of when he had entered the country.

Every month or two Aaron's voice would greet me on the phone. My first reaction was always pleasure, no matter how

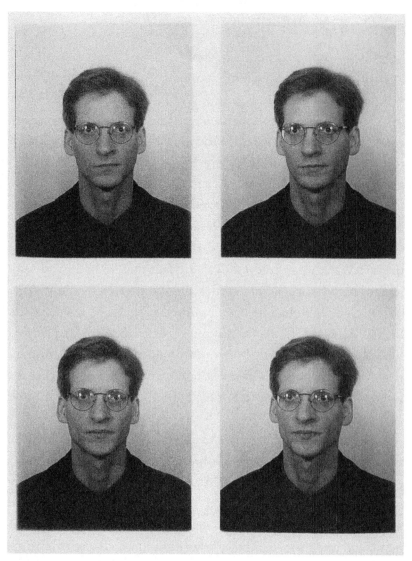

Aaron's self-portrait, Paris, 1995

difficult the conversation that followed. He might chat about Paris or a town he was visiting. Or he might be angry. Often enough he brought up his idea that I wasn't his mother.

"Aaron, I'm your mother."

"That's what you say."

"Why else would I go through this?"

"Maybe you're being paid."

Paid to pretend, paid to cooperate with the people who watched him and followed him and imitated him, who knew his thoughts and insulted him out loud, who told television newscasters to speak directly to him, who singled him out for torment. Paid, evidently, all his life, to invent the story of his birth and tell it to him every year.

I found a source of hope in news stories about John Forbes Nash Jr. (who was no relation to any Forbes in Arthur's family). Nash had recently won a Nobel Prize for his work in game theory. What interested me was the fact that he had lived with schizophrenia for several decades and spontaneously returned to sanity. Only then had he been honored with the Nobel for work he had done before his breakdown. Chris Beels confirmed that such things do happen. For some time I clung to the thought that Aaron's illness might eventually run its course. By then he would have lost many years of his life—but he would be himself again, or more himself.

He was never far from my thoughts. The model sailboat he and Arthur had made stood silhouetted against the window, a good forty inches from the keel to the top of the mast. On my desk lay the envelope containing his most recent note, so I could see his name and his *poste restante* address in the corner, and my name and our address, all neatly written in his all-capitals printing.

As the spring semester began at Baruch, everyone in the Department of Academic Skills was talking about Governor Pataki's proposed cuts to CUNY. People expected the department to be eliminated, and anxiety about jobs ran high. I was worried too. I didn't want to lose this position a short walk from home where my supervisors were congenial and my students well-prepared.

To deal with my anxiety, and because I enjoyed taking a stand, I threw myself into organizing protests, joining with other faculty and staff across CUNY. I told my students about Pataki's proposals. If a protest was scheduled for our class time, I invited them to attend with me. Before we went, I handed out poster board and markers so they could write placards.

Reality hit when I received the college president's letter for the following semester. In one sentence I was told I would have no job in the fall.

Around this time 311 had its first inspection by the city as part of our efforts to bring the building up to code. As the architect and I walked the inspector through the house, he found esoteric and expensive violations. He called off the inspection halfway through, leaving us without a complete list of problems to be corrected.

"He wants you to pay him off," the architect told me. But I wasn't willing to do that.

I had lost my job. Now my house was threatened, throwing me into a state of frantic insecurity. Reason told me I would save myself a lot of headaches by selling the house and living somewhere else. But I couldn't. Instead I clung to my exoskeleton, an integral part of me, not a sheddable shell.

Again I felt alone with my predicament. I reasoned that the house was my problem, not Arthur's, though he and I still shared joint ownership. He came downtown now and then to deal with a plumber or an inspector and did the bookkeeping for our taxes. I could hardly expect more of him. Though Jay lived in the house with me, I excluded him too from responsibility. After all, he was working full-time. While he was always willing to shovel snow or run down to the hardware store for a radiator valve, he couldn't share my feeling about 311. It was comfortable, but hermit crabs aren't picky. So would plenty of other places be. I struggled along on my own.

Home for my fiftieth birthday in June, Stasha had a short haircut and new glasses she had spent obsessive weeks choosing. But she couldn't stop belittling me, even when we had friends over to celebrate my birthday.

"Stasha, you put me down so much," I told her next day.

"I do?"

"You do. Think of how you were talking about me at my party."

"I feel bad," she said. "And upset." She seemed close to tears.

"Do you want to go for a walk?" I thought it would be easier to talk if we could get out of the house.

"OK." We went down to Saint Mark's Churchyard, a little patch of trees and gravestones on 10th Street. As traffic coursed down Second Avenue, we seated ourselves awkwardly on a burial stone. I put an arm around Stasha.

"I love you," I said.

She started to cry. "I'll try not to say those things now I know you love me."

I was stricken by her words. What had I done wrong that my daughter didn't know I loved her? She was touchy, dubious about her competence—so much so that when a volunteer job helping at a film festival had produced a job offer, she had turned it down. Now she was thinking of another volunteer position.

"You might feel better if you had a paying job," I said.

"You're always telling me what you think I should do."

"Stasha, I love you. I love you *soooo* much." I added our special gesture from her childhood, holding my hands apart to show how enormous my love for her was. I realized I needed to remind her often. It had been better, it seemed to me, when she had lived with us. I had enjoyed her presence more and been able to support her better.

When Aaron called, he often demanded I stop what was happening to him. Too often I told him that only medication would stop it.

"You want me to see a psychiatrist. Dr. White ignored me. He was consciously intending to do what he did. Everything was by design, from his name to where we met. Dr. Goff was an ambitious, mediocre doctor, willing to put patients through abusive experiments."

I had no idea what Aaron believed White had done "by design," but I was sure it wasn't worth pursuing.

"Why did you get the diagnosis of schizophrenia from Dr. Goff?" I asked.

"I didn't have money. I went to Dr. Goff and pretended to be crazy to get disability. I'm not crazy. I'm not psychotic, whatever you believe. But you're in a position to make things better."

"If I were, they wouldn't have happened the way they did."

My helplessness made me angry at myself. The worm of self-reproach never slept.

Over the summer I was again teaching at Baruch and dashing off for interviews all over New York. I still didn't have a job in August when Jay and I made our first trip to Maine to stay in a tent on the lawn of my cousins Weslea and Curtis. Wes is connected to me through our Blaufarb grandfathers; her resemblance to my Blaufarb aunts is one of the pleasure of being friends with her.

Jay and I drank our morning coffee on Curtis and Weslea's porch, then drove off to explore each morning. In Acadia National Park we climbed the well-made rock steps of Mount Dorr, breathing the fragrant pine, strengthened by the mountain's great bulwarks of granite. On the bare summit a thousand feet up, we sat down by a patch of pines bent close to the rock. The wind sang gently over the mountain. The vast Atlantic lay before us, its blue almost merging with the blue of the sky. We decided that next summer we would find a place near here.

Calling home for my messages, I found one from the English Department at Baruch. Did I want to teach a combined reading and writing course for advanced ESL students? I called right back to say I did.

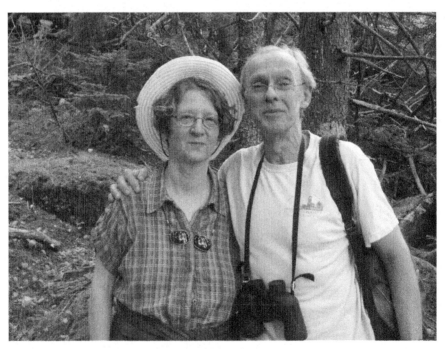

Ingrid and Jay, Mount Dorr, Maine, 2012

And in September, on our third try, the house passed the Buildings Department inspection, conducted now by a different inspector, and we were granted a new Certificate of Occupancy. But after calling every bank I could think of, I couldn't find one that would give us a mortgage. There seemed no solution—we would have to sell the house. When I went to the credit union to tell the director we would be selling, lo and behold!—the policy on commercial mortgages had changed and we were now eligible.

Within weeks my practical dilemmas had been solved. I had my home, I had a job. Outwardly my life was more settled and secure than it had been for years. My sense of gloom, of loss, of precariousness hung on.

The ups of Aaron's illness were the rare moments when he seemed more like himself—articulate, sensible, free of anger. Mostly there were downs and more downs. My bitterness was a seething, grating, raw misery, which intensified when he pleaded again that I stop what I was doing to him. My distress seeped into my attitudes toward my friends, who were tactless and self-involved, and toward Jay, who was unbearably vulnerable. "Aaron's illness changes everything," I had told Ellen Wachtel years earlier. It did.

Seeing my state, my therapist suggested I try an antidepressant. A year earlier, with a prescription from my internist, I had begun with too strong a dose and soon found myself sick with headache and nausea. This time Chris Beels gave me a schedule for gradually building up the dosage. And this time the medication worked. Within a few weeks my rancor abated. It didn't disappear, but it wasn't so acute. My friends might be self-centered, but they were also kind, and Jay was vulnerable but intelligent and helpful.

In San Francisco, Stasha was gradually coming undone. "It's not right for me to be able to do what I want when Aaron can't," she told me once. She had given up looking for work and wouldn't take a temporary job. For a time she would barely talk on the phone. More commonly, she called me several times a day with little questions. On Thanksgiving she dished out meals at a soup kitchen. The week before her thirtieth birthday in February, she was overwhelmed with a sense of crisis. She bought a plane ticket home, and I found myself hoping she would stay on with me and Jay. It was too hard to support her from a distance. She had the same idea.

"I'm not going back," she said, when she had come in and shed her parka and let me give her something to eat.

"Good," I said. "You can stay with us."

"I need to figure out what I'm going to do and then I'll find myself an apartment."

So Stasha took over the little room Jay had been using, ousting his belongings piece by piece.

This was all fine with me. It was harder for Jay. Sometimes we upset him with our wrangling. Other times we outvoted him about videos to watch.

"I feel like moving out," he said crankily one evening when it was just the two of us at dinner. His tone told me this was a protest, rather than a plan. I flared up indignantly.

"You feel like moving out. My son is psychotic, my daughter is depressed, and you feel like moving out." I got up and left him alone at the table.

Before long he presented his contrite face at the bedroom door. "I feel like an idiot," he said.

"You were an idiot, but it's OK. I'll forgive you," I said, half

joking at my own magnanimity. At times I too felt pressed. I
wanted to support Stasha and often enjoyed her presence. But
responding to her moodiness and her needs could seem like
another contraction of Ingridity.

After Jay's outburst, he and I and Stasha had a session or two
with Ellen Wachtel to think about our newly increased household.

"I think this is what both of you need," Ellen said, addressing
me and Stasha. "You've both been wanting family. These days
a lot of grown kids return to live with their parents. It's not
unusual." With Ellen's encouragement, we worked out how to
reorganize our apartment.

Jay decided to rent space at the Writers Room on nearby Astor
Place. He marked student work wherever he could find a spot in
the house—at my desk in the bedroom or the kitchen table.

In one of my sporadic fits of straightening up, I grumbled at
Stasha. "I don't want those Bean catalogs piling up on the coffee
table."

"I hate it when you're in this mood," she said matter-of-
factly, making Jay laugh, rather too sympathetically, I thought.

Together Stasha and I made a plan to visit Paris over my spring
break. Happily, Aaron was pleased by the idea.

"Do you think I should look for an apartment?" he asked.

"If that's what you want."

"Could you help me when you visit?"

"We can talk about that when we get there."

"I haven't been very organized. I don't know if I'm present-
able. I haven't been able to make calls about an apartment or go
into a realtor's office. My courage fails me," he said, rather
heartbreakingly. But I didn't pause to be sad, I was so excited

that he was welcoming us, so happy I would see him after eighteen months. I called friends for guidance on apartment hunting in Paris. Stasha and I met with Chris Beels and planned our trip, though I remained nervous that Aaron would find some reason to refuse to see us.

We reached Paris on a damp spring morning, found the Hotel Capucines on the hill of Montmartre, and collapsed on the two narrow beds in our room. The phone woke us.

"*Il y a un homme pour vous, madame,*" the proprietor said.

"*C'est mon fils,*" I told her. How good it felt to say that: it's my son. As I opened our door to him, I impulsively took his hand and kissed it, and got a disgusted look. But he leaned over Stasha, who was sitting up on the bed, and kissed her. As he sat in the straight chair by the window, I examined him. His hair was very short, his clothes were neat, he was not too pale, not too thin. But he had a way of jerking his head back a little and rolling his eyes to the side, as if listening for meaning behind our words, I thought. His cheeks were sunken by the tension in his face. My pleasure in being with him was eroded by his discomfort.

"What are your plans?" he asked.

"We came to see you."

"I need to eat," Stasha said, rousing herself from the bed.

"OK. We'll go out. Would you like to have lunch with us?" I asked Aaron.

"I'm not hungry."

"You can sit with us."

Outside in the gray and damp air, we walked uphill to the shops and cafés on the rue des Abbesses. Stasha chose a little luncheonette and I ordered for us, using my basic but serviceable French. Grimacing, Aaron refused everything but a coffee. His voice tense and clipped, he asked what Arthur was doing.

"Arthur's painting a lot," I told him. "And taking photographs."

Arthur's mother had died the previous spring. Now Aaron asked about her will, which he had obtained from J.M. Forbes as a beneficiary and read with care. He asked whether Arthur and I would change our financial package to him.

"Are you living with Ingrid, Stasha?"

She nodded and began to cry at his strained and angry manner.

"Are you studying acting?" he asked, to discount her distress.

On the street, he scolded us for spending too much on lunch. He was used to managing on so little.

"When would you like to go apartment hunting?" I asked. "I've done some homework."

"I don't want to look," he said.

"Aaron, you want an apartment. Let's at least make an effort."

"No. There's no use. It isn't possible to find one. "

"I insist on trying. What about the American Church? They have listings."

"They have eight or ten a day. But I don't want to go there."

"What about looking in the paper for ads?"

"No, Ingrid. I don't want to. Don't do it."

My excitement at the chance to help prevented me from adjusting to his change of mind. So he made one of his angry exits, striding off down the narrow street as we stood helplessly by. But I didn't despair of seeing him again. We would be in Paris another five days.

Stasha and I walked around Montmartre, gazing through the windows of bakeries and butchers, then took the *métro* to the American Church and copied apartment listings—until I took in that what we were doing made no sense.

Next morning Aaron called, still upset. He refused to see us though he must have been nearby: I could hear the blaring loud-speakers of the rue des Abbesses merchants on his end of the line.

"I don't want an apartment. I've decided against it. You and Arthur have to have my agreement before you start looking for me."

"Right. I've changed my mind. I won't look for an apartment if you don't want me to."

He went over his Visa bill. Would we pay it off? Though the Visa debt was his mistake, his mistakes were our mistakes since he was dependent on us, he explained. He went over other financial details, and I wondered unhappily if he planned not to see us again.

With no way to get hold of Aaron, we spent our time exploring the city. Stasha was good at figuring out the *métro* and went off into peals of infectious laughter at her own silliness. Sharing our little room, enjoying croissants and café au lait each morning in the hotel dining room, roaming the city during the day, she and I hadn't been together so much for years. We held each other a lot and kissed good night before we went to sleep. During the days we crisscrossed the city, passing under the Seine in the *métro*, walking across it, taking a boat ride down it, passing under an ancient bridge. We walked through the Tuileries and rode a bus past the Bastille. The Bastille! I was excited.

Visiting Mexico City with Jay over Christmas just a few months earlier, I had been too depressed to enjoy myself. Despite the richness of Mexican history and its pre-Columbian and post-Columbian art, I had been disturbed by the losses and pain of the conquest, visible throughout the city, and the poverty that was its legacy. My energy had been low, and I kept having to stop for a coffee or a meal. On this trip I found I had the stamina to get through the day; it was Stasha who often needed a break for a snack or a rest. Buoyed by the medication I was

168

taking, and perhaps by being in the same city as Aaron, and despite the chilly damp, I felt a wonderful release from my narrow daily round of teaching and landlady chores, the blinkered regimen I had imposed on myself. The shock of freedom was so dramatic that it was frightening. I woke one night from a dream that Stasha and I had accidentally freed a woman who had been imprisoned underground, calling out in my sleep as if I were an ambulance alarm.

"Mom, Mom, Mom," Stasha was saying as she shook my shoulder.

As the date for our flight back home neared, I worried that Aaron wouldn't call again. But on the morning of our last day, he phoned the hotel.

"Aaron, I'd like to see you before we leave. Why don't you have supper with us tonight?"

"No, I'm busy."

"But we came all this way. I hate to leave without seeing you again."

"I'm tired. I don't want to."

"I have something I want to give you, a little memento."

"OK. I'll meet you at the hotel at eight."

Stasha and I lingered over our meal at a restaurant near the hotel till it was time for her to return to meet Aaron. Before long the two of them came in, and Aaron sat down next to me, which in itself was remarkable. Unwilling to let us order him a meal, he agreed to finish up Stasha's generous platter. He peeled the paper from the little box that contained his gift, bought in Mexico before I knew we would make this visit. It was a thimble of mother-of-pearl and red enamel, which I had chosen because it was charming and because I knew Aaron used a thimble when he sewed. Taking it from the box, he smiled. He was so pleased that he smiled as he put the thimble on his forefinger.

"It fits," he said. "I'll use it. I have to shorten a pair of pants." He put it in his pocket. "I've been going through a process of reassessment. There are a lot of things that don't make sense in my life. I know you think that's because I have a mental illness."

"I do." I also thought that his process of reassessment was part of his paranoia.

"Tell me one thing that suggests it," he said.

For a moment I was silent, searching for an answer to his question that wouldn't antagonize him. "You think I'm not your mother."

"I can't defend myself."

"I *am* your mother."

"It would be terrible if you weren't."

To me it seemed terrible that he often believed what was painful to him.

"If you took medication and were in treatment, you could work. You wouldn't be so isolated."

"I don't think so." He couldn't imagine that. "I don't know anyone in the States except you and Stasha and Arthur."

"That's a pretty good support system," Stasha said, speaking, I thought, of her own experience.

"How have you been spending your time?" he asked.

"Sightseeing. Paris seems like a nice city."

"That wears off after a few months."

"What do you want to do about an apartment?" I asked.

"The listings at the American Church are mostly prostitutes or call girls. If you don't believe me, call yourself. The things they say don't make sense." Another of his delusions. "I'm afraid that if I signed a lease it would become a nightmare and then I'd be stuck." So that was why he didn't want an apartment.

"What do you want to do?" I asked. But he didn't know what he wanted.

He let me kiss him good-bye, and Stasha walked him to the *métro*.

"He looks so crazy," she said, meeting me on the steps of the hotel. "As he walked down the *métro* steps, he had his head on one side and his eyes were rolling a little."

Still we were jubilant, crowing and laughing as we went up to our room. For an hour and a half Aaron had sat quietly with us, his tone friendly and calm. It was years now since he had been so amiable. With much excitement we called Arthur and Jay to report on our success, then packed our bags for our flight in the morning.

I knew it was good luck that Aaron's frame of mind had allowed him to meet with us, when he had refused to see Arthur for more than fifteen minutes a few months earlier. It was no more than chance that I had a gift for him, and that my mention of it persuaded him to see us. Or perhaps he was beginning a period of remission, though we saw no more signs of this for another year.

That summer Jay and I rented a little cabin in Maine, on the mainland not far from Weslea and Curtis. After a long day of driving, we found our way to Patten Pond late at night and fell asleep to the sound of loons calling on the pond. When we woke we found ourselves a few feet from the pond, as Mainers often call a lake. The loons were swimming low in the water, then diving and surfacing a minute or two later in another spot.

We quickly fell into a rhythm of days of writing, hiking, cooking. Evenings we listened to audiobooks of Agatha Christie mysteries, and enjoyed occasional dinners out with Curtis and Weslea. After supper we would often drive fifteen minutes to the pebble beach on Union Bay. Sitting on the dark stones worn by the ocean into terraces, we would watch the clouds overhead change colors in the setting sun and admire the mountains across the water on Mount Desert Island, their spines forming the eastern horizon. Jay would lift his binoculars to watch an osprey plummet down after a fish, or more often to sight a cormorant or a duck. I might take a thread of dried seaweed to tickle Jay lightly on the back of his neck until he swatted at what he thought was a mosquito, then turned, his eyes brightening, his laugh joining mine.

My project was the memoir I had begun, focusing on my relationship with my father. Jay's novel was more fantasy than science fiction, he told me. He set up his computer on the screened porch, which allowed him to keep on eye out for wildlife nearby. Several times a day he would grab his binoculars and go out to investigate the doings on the pond or in the thicket near the house. His gossip concerned the birds. "The mother loon is on the lake," he told me when he returned from outside. "One of the chicks keeps trying to get on her back. He's at least half her size, so all he can do is rub at her back with his bill. She pushes him away, and he tries her from the other side." Or, after a riot of squawking and cawing in the pines, he would report on the jays. Once or twice he paddled off at daybreak in an old canoe so he could fish, coming home with small perch or bass he gutted and cleaned and cooked.

Our favorite hike was twenty minutes from the camp up "our mountain," known to the world as Great Pond Mountain. We would go anytime of day to climb to the pink granite summit, rounded off by the ice of the last glaciers. From the top we would check out the views of the surrounding hills and the coast. Sometimes we would even go after supper, clambering up in the dusk and descending through the near dark to bump our rented car slowly down the gravel road to Route 1.

Before bed on moonless nights, I would wrap myself in a quilt and we would feel our way in the dark across the grass and up the slope, guided by the lighter patches of sky between the dark masses of the pines. In the field I would throw my head back to gaze across the millennia at the brilliance of the Milky Way arcing across the sky.

Chapter 13

A year later, in August of 1997, Aaron decided to come home. Arthur phoned me in Maine with the news.

"He called you? He's coming back?"

"Yes. That's what he said."

"Did he say when?"

"Maybe next week, as soon as he can get a ticket."

I was excited. It was more than a year since Stasha and I had seen Aaron in Paris. But what did it mean that he was returning? Was he going to make one of his brief appearances and then vanish again? Would he go back to Boston? I didn't imagine he would stay with us after his years of distance.

Jay and I spent our last day packing and cleaning and loading the car with our suitcases and duffel bags of clothes and bedding and boxes of books and notebooks till we could just see over the heaps in the backseat. The first few hours of the long trip home took us through Maine pines. As we skirted the urban sprawl between Boston and Worcester, Massachusetts, the traffic grew denser, and my anticipation of seeing Aaron after fifteen months grew stronger, along with my nervousness. By Connecticut we could feel New York City's centripetal pull sucking us in, the arteries flowing with vehicles of every description. Then Manhattan and the energy of being almost home, the familiar miles following the East River, till we were on city streets, threading our way to the door. As we got out of the rental car to haul our belongings into the house, we found our neighbor, José, on our stoop. "I saw Aaron," he said.

And once we got upstairs, there he was, sitting on the couch as if it were the most natural thing in the world. He glanced up, his face more relaxed, more like himself, as I thought, than when we had seen him in Paris. He greeted us and asked about our trip, chatted, and showed no signs of restlessness, no indication he wanted to leave.

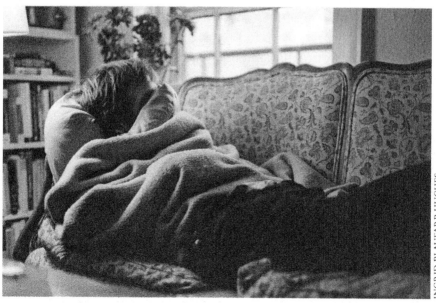

Aaron on the couch at Ingrid's, 1997

Next morning Stasha and I brought him up-to-date on our neighbors.

"José got married," I told Aaron. José was rather prickly, as he himself readily acknowledged.

"Really?"

"Yes, his wife is a teacher. She seems nice. He says she was reduced to marrying him by the man shortage. There just aren't enough marriageable men, according to him."

"The man shortage." Aaron smiled.

"José is funny," Stasha said.

After the years of our separation, how intensely sweet it was to be sitting on a quiet Sunday morning in my living room with both my children, chuckling over an amusing bit of gossip. Aaron seemed so ordinary, quite free of paranoia or derision. For a moment I allowed myself to hope that this mood would prevail.

But no. Aaron would talk to me, but he would rarely let me put a hand on his arm or give him a hug. "Don't touch me. Fuck off. Don't sit near me." He still believed I was pretending to be his mother, and Arthur and I were joining with others to interfere in his life and make him miserable.

At times he seemed hunched and frail. For no apparent reason he might lift his arms, as if to protect himself from a blow. He came and went at all hours, often visiting Arthur and Lanie, and slept his irregular sleep on the living room couch. He washed his few items of clothing by hand, hanging his socks and underwear to dry on a lampshade. He was distant with Stasha, more talkative with Jay, and rather sweet with our aging cat, Felicity. "Felicity and I have an understanding," he told me. She was one of our few safe topics.

Sometimes he helped himself to one of my soups from the stove, or even sat down with us for a meal, satisfying my deep instinct to feed my child. He took pictures of me washing dishes at the kitchen sink, which I interpreted as an act of affection. Though living with him was bruising, I was glad to have him nearby, tall, thin, handsome, broad-shouldered.

I was teaching now at Bronx Community College, way up past Yankee Stadium, on a breezy hill that looked west all the way to the Jersey Palisades. My students were almost all from the Dominican Republic, social and agreeable and usually female.

Downtown I was at the Borough of Manhattan Community College, near the World Trade Center. Twice a week I dashed off to BMCC for an 8:00 a.m. reading class with twenty-five incoming freshmen. They were mainstream students just graduated from city high schools who resented having to take a remedial course and were prone to backtalk. One morning I heard myself responding to a minor piece of impertinence from a student with tit for her tat, something I scorned and would not ordinarily fall into. It was Aaron I was bickering with, I realized. Living with his hostility was affecting my relations with my students.

At first he bounced between 311 and Arthur and Lanie's apartment on West 85th Street as he pleased. But soon Arthur asked if Aaron could live with us, pointing out that we had two bedrooms to his and Lanie's one. We also had three people in our two bedrooms, so this argument wasn't strong. I supposed that Lanie wasn't comfortable with Aaron, and Jay was, if not comfortable, accommodating. Though I didn't think of denying Arthur's request, it was wearing to have both my children living with us. The apartment seemed congested, with piles of books and teaching folders and the *New York Times* on the coffee table. On my desk my landlady checkbook in its three-ring binder waited for me to work my way through the monthly bills. Aaron was often stretched out on the couch. His little pack stood in a corner. Arthur called often, worrying about Aaron, suggesting ways to deal with him, which were not always practical. It wasn't until the break provided by the Jewish holidays in October that I got my boxes from Maine unpacked and dug out my winter work clothes.

I had left Arthur seven years earlier when my children were in their twenties, off leading their own lives. Now they were living with me again, and I talked to Arthur often about Aaron. I felt disoriented. In my sleep I was with Arthur and he was leaving me, rather than the other way around. I was with Jay in a great storm and I couldn't see where we lived.

Awake, I moved through my days dealing with the tasks immediately before me: going over student work and planning for the next day's class, running out to buy groceries when the fridge was empty, picking up take-out on my way home if I didn't want to cook. I was grateful for the falafel place on Second Avenue, and the combination platter of pierogis and stuffed cabbage at Veselka.

When Aaron got in touch with Katherine, they resumed the romance that had broken off during their college years. With her he was so much himself that I wondered if she could understand how serious his illness was. She came to visit one weekend, as slender as always, the long hair of her teens now cropped close to her head, revealing a long neck.

"What's going on with you?" I asked her. We had stayed in touch and I knew she had completed her master's in education in the spring.

"I'm teaching fourth grade up in Washington Heights."

"Fourth grade? That's a great age."

"Yes. It's a great age. My favorite age. I've always wanted to teach fourth grade. But they're bouncing off the walls. We didn't study classroom management at Harvard."

Katherine had an apartment not far from the school where she was teaching. Because her new job was so demanding, she rarely let Aaron spend the night with her during the week. He pleaded with her daily to let him stay, until she called me in distress.

"You sound terrible," I told her. "Do you have a cold?"

"No, I'm hoarse from yelling at my class. I don't know what to say to Aaron. He keeps begging me to let him sleep here."

"Just be firm," I said. "Tell him he can't keep asking, it's too hard on you."

Katherine called again a few days later to see if I had told Aaron she should put him up, as he claimed. Of course, I hadn't. Then he said he would see a psychiatrist if she gave in. This worked until he confessed he had no intention of keeping his promise. All of which he told me when he reappeared at 311, bringing in a little Entenmann's pie, eating it, and getting straight into the bath.

Aaron's lies to Katherine, his unashamed confession of them, his nastiness to me reveal a childlike morality—which shows that our morality comes out of our experience. His experience was a world made up of lies, a reality of manipulations and cruelties which everyone around him denied. Lying was the only way he could get what he needed.

If Katherine was too stressed from her teaching to deal with him, I was his scapegoat. His hostility became a deliberate strategy when he convinced himself that Katherine would take him in if he harassed me so much I threw him out. He spent two evenings raging at me, threatening to pack up my books because, he said, "They're all feminist and all by women."

Glancing at the bookshelves where the three fat volumes of
À la recherche du temps perdu were conspicuous, I asked,
"What about Proust?"

"Proust was a woman," he said crankily, and continued his
diatribe. As he scolded me, I reminded myself that growing up
he had never seen a reason to question feminism or call a gay
man a woman.

At six the next morning, he opened our bedroom door and
started in again. I slid out of bed so Jay could sleep, and Aaron
followed me to the kitchen to continue his harangue while I
drank coffee.

When I could talk to Chris Beels later in the day, he fortified
me. I took his advice.

"Aaron, you can't stay here if you're going to insult me all the
time."

"I wouldn't insult you if you weren't such a man-hating feminist."

"That's the kind of thing I mean. It's not OK."

"Say that as if you mean it."

This wasn't my Aaron. At times like this I could understand
the idea of a dybbuk, the malicious spirit of Jewish folklore that
takes over a person and talks with his voice.

Often Aaron would stretch out on the couch, his large head at
one end, his large feet at the other, pull up the wool overcoat he
had bought at a thrift shop, and lie muttering into the back of
the couch. "The point being . . ." he would begin and go on
about what was wrong with Arthur or me.

"I can't hear you," I would say and say again. So conscien-
tious a communicator am I that it took me a while to see that it
was easier to let him mutter on unheard than to respond to his

diatribes. He'd start on education, maybe, which was what he had loved, till his illness made it impossible. Now teachers were self-serving, like doctors, the subject of another monologue.

Once, as I sat with a pile of student papers, he questioned me about a cousin whose academic career had fizzled when he didn't get tenure. This led directly to his own experience of a malevolent academia. Since he had obviously not been good enough to be at MIT, he must have been accepted because a Forbes—"some genetic supremacist"—wanted to pay MIT to take him. The comprehensive exams he had passed as his last effort had been rigged in his favor. And what about my "sinister father" and Arthur's "sinister background"? (By this he meant the Forbes history in the China trade.) Had the CIA and the Forbeses colluded to arrange our marriage? Or had I married Arthur for his money?

As Aaron expatiated on these ideas, I made brief answers, or sat silent, my red pen laid aside, a student essay half read on my lap. But I did rouse myself to correct his final point. "No, I did *not* marry Arthur for his money," I said firmly, and probably a bit indignantly.

Aaron lay back and pulled his blanket over his face. By evening he wouldn't talk to me at all. The advantage of this was that it allowed me to finish my correcting without more distractions, since Jay was teaching.

Stasha too was out, attending a class in early childhood education at City College. Before long she got work as an occasional substitute at a nearby nursery school. It was good to see her mood lift on the days when she worked.

Often I attended meetings of adjuncts from a number of CUNY campuses, working to improve our pay and working conditions. We traded stories of department offices shared sometimes by forty or fifty of us in and out of one room over the course of a week. We complained about our invisibility to full-timers. We taught each other about the few rights the union contract provided us and strategized to enlarge our role in the union of CUNY faculty and staff. We carried union application cards around with us, talking to adjuncts on our campuses whenever we had a chance. Our work together offered far more immediate satisfaction than sitting in a room by myself to write a book. In my organizing there was always the reinforcement of relationships to carry me on. Along with my teaching, it provided a focus for my life outside our family, and away from the pain of living with Aaron.

At home I'm afraid I took for granted Jay's ability to accept Aaron as part of our household. Though Jay seemed uneasy and even at times outright uncomfortable, I persuaded myself this was because he was teaching a different level this year and his classes met five days a week, rather than the usual four. On a Saturday morning, when Aaron was at Katherine's and Stasha sleeping in, we had a rare moment alone over our coffee.

"I dreamt I was getting married to a younger man," I told him. "The wedding consisted of me standing up and making a pronouncement." (How like me, with my assertions and pronouncements.)

Jay laughed. "We could get married. Why don't we?" he said. But if my dream suggested marriage, awake I wasn't ready. The pleasures of our summer had faded; my energies were dispersed.

Then Aaron's restlessness carried him away again. "I'm going in November. I have my ticket. I may stay away a long time," he told me.

And then I didn't want him to leave. While he was bathing, I zipped his backpack open to look at his bus ticket. El Paso, Texas. At least he would remain in the country.

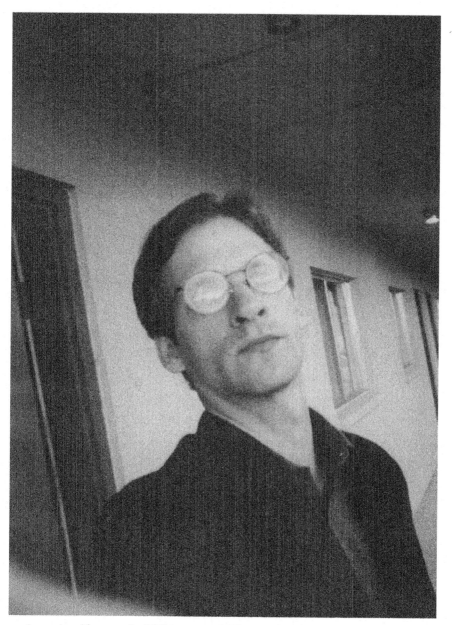

Aaron's self-portrait, El Paso motel, Texas, 1998

———

In March Aaron turned up at Arthur's, worried about his health and wanting a referral to an internist. He also wanted to see a dentist. Over the next year, the year preceding his death, he saw a number of doctors for various reasons—I think now, because he expected to live and wanted to take care of himself. At the same time he was thinking about dying. He told me he had wished his plane would crash on his flight from El Paso. "But unfortunately it didn't." Arthur mentioned his remarks about a shortened life span.

Another sign of health was his return to the family. He had ended his isolation of five years in Boston and France and come back to us, then gone off to Texas and found his way home again after just a few months. Despite his sometime belief that we weren't his parents, he acted as if we were. For that I was grateful. But I never forgot that he had been another person before he got sick.

I too had been another person. I knew now at the deepest level the truth we work so hard to deny: we don't always control our own lives, though good fortune lets us think we do and hard luck makes us want to believe we can do anything we set our minds to. All our can-do attitudes can't protect us from illness and accidents, wars, tornadoes, societal cruelties. Understanding that, I had more empathy for others in pain, more humility, a larger humanity.

While I was perhaps wiser, I was also shaken to my core. I could no longer believe I was the wonderful mother I used to think myself. My children's sorrows hurt my ability to love myself. Though I wrote over the summers, my pride in my writing was faltering too. My novel sat in a box on a shelf. In the past I had submitted poems and stories indefatigably, willing to receive dozens of rejections for every piece published in a literary journal. Now I lacked the stamina for that kind of relentless effort. Fulfilling my responsibilities as a teacher, a mother, a landlady, I slogged on.

A day or two after returning to Arthur's, Aaron stopped by 311 for his mail.

"I haven't seen you for months. You can stay for a bit. Just sit down. Do you want something to eat?" I said.

He put down his backpack. "Do you have any fruit?"

"I do. Lots," I said, feeling well provisioned. I put together a fruit salad. For the moment, Aaron was willing to eat the food I prepared, to sit at the table without insulting me. I was happy for any moment of peace between us.

"I'm worried about parasites," he told me. "I used to go over the bridge to Mexico every day. Customs used to ask me the reason for my visit. I always told them lunch."

A few days later he came by again. "I got my lab results. No parasites, no amoebas. Cleanest shit this side of the Mississippi." I laughed.

Stasha came in and he repeated his good news; they agreed to go out to Veselka for coffee. "Although I don't think you need to eat," he said. "You're fat enough."

"I'm not going out with you if you talk that way."

"You hurt Stasha's feelings," I said, as though Aaron were a small child.

"I'm sorry, Stash. I shouldn't have said that."

"Aaron doesn't usually apologize," I pointed out to Stasha.

"I'm not very good at feelings," he said.

"OK. Next subject," Stasha said, a phrase we often used to conclude a topic. And they went out.

Whenever the two of them found a way to be together for a little while, I was pleased. Often they coexisted uneasily; occasionally a bitter squabble blew up, as if they were ten and twelve again. Aaron wanted to be friends with Stasha, with Katherine, with his high school friend, Miranda. But I was sadly aware that his friendships would always be limited by his illness. It took a strong bond to put up with Aaron's obstreperousness.

"He isn't charming," I told Chris Beels.

"Schizophrenics aren't," he said.

Again Katherine told Aaron he could live with her if he would see a psychiatrist. This time he made an appointment with a doctor whose name we got from Chris Beels.

"Do you think I should trust Katherine?" Aaron asked. "What if she goes back on her word and doesn't let me live with her even if I take medication?"

"I think she'll do what she promised to do."

He kept his appointment, informed us that he liked the doctor, and filled the prescription she gave him.

"I've never seen anything come of this kind of deal," Chris Beels said.

I thought it was unlikely myself. Aaron had been living with his illness for years now. While he often chafed at the way his life was and restlessly sought out new situations, he didn't believe medication would help. As Chris pointed out, his distrust of doctors worked against his acceptance of their prescriptions. Still, despite the stoicism I had developed in dealing with Aaron, I couldn't help feeling a bit hopeful.

A month later Aaron saw the psychiatrist again to tell her the medication had been effective without his taking a single dose, because it had made Katherine take him in.

"I don't need to see a psychiatrist. I'm not delusional," he said.
"No?"

"I'm not," he said. "Other people think I am."

"But you complain that your life is limited."

"It is limited." But his illness had so completely taken him in that he couldn't remember or imagine the Aaron we thought the real one.

Several times I found myself dreaming that Aaron had AIDS, perhaps because I understood at some level well below consciousness that his illness might prove fatal. Like AIDS, it was stigmatized and frightening to people. Like AIDS, it required extensive support, a team of friends and doctors. Like AIDS, it was devastating and incurable and often hit young men. But increasingly, in the nineties, AIDS could be lived with if a person took medication, as schizophrenia could—though like Aaron, people with AIDS and HIV didn't always do that.

While Aaron was staying with Arthur for a few days, Stasha played happily with Felicity, picking her up, cradling her, saying, "Felicity has something to tell you."

"What?"

"She says she loves you." It was wonderful to see Stasha happy. During the rare moments when Stasha and Aaron both seemed well, I thought maybe I would be able to live my life after all— by which I meant pursue my writing with more energy.

On the wide sidewalk outside Herman Badillo's office, I marched in circles with other faculty and students, chanting *"Abajo, Badillo"* and *"El pueblo unido jamás sera vencido."* The students' energy was contagious, and I enjoyed the directness of their slogans.

They held up placards saying BADILLO, THE BUTCHER OF CUNY and BADILLO, ENEMY OF THE PEOPLE. As chairman of the City University's Board of Trustees, Badillo was leading attacks on open admissions. His plan was to cut remediation from the system's senior colleges, forcing students who needed developmental courses into the community colleges.

I agreed with the students: narrowing access would choke off the best route out of hardship and poverty for many of the two hundred thousand enrolled at CUNY campuses. Whether our protests succeeded or not, I wanted to stand publicly in support of open admissions on every campus.

At Bronx Community a student came to class wiping tears from her eyes with her neat pastel sleeve. Welfare had told her she had to withdraw from her courses—a woman with three children and a mother to support, sentenced to sweeping parks by President Clinton's cuts in welfare benefits. Another student couldn't go to a protest scheduled to follow our class for lack of a dollar for the subway. That was easy to fix: I bought him two tokens, and we took the train together. On East 80th Street outside the CUNY Board of Trustees meeting, we joined seven or eight hundred protesters. While we stood vigil, the Board of Trustees was voting to restrict admissions. Bitter and sad, I knew it was exactly my students who would suffer. Immigrants, women, and students of color were most likely to need remediation, most likely to be already balancing work, family, and school.

Jay was visiting family out west at Passover. Katherine had left for a week in Paris with her sister, and Aaron was gloomy. Stasha and I got together a meal of lamb, matzo, and haroset, pot-roasting the lamb with vegetables and lemon to produce a rich sauce for the tender meat. The three of us loaded our plates and seated

ourselves in the living room to eat from our laps, telling ourselves we were reclining like free people. That was the extent of
our celebration of the festival of freedom.

"Now what?" Aaron asked, staring off at the wall of books he
had complained were all feminist. "When you're thirty, you're
supposed to accept your lot in life. It's hard when it's so incredibly miniscule."

"Does it have to be that way?" I asked, thinking of medication. But there was no sense bringing that up.

"Yes."

"Are you sure?"

"I'm pretty certain," he said. "Though I hope. The problem is
there's no significance to anything I can do."

Aaron was right. His lot was narrow. We all had to live with
that. I concentrated on eating my lamb and crunching my matzo.

The studio on the second floor came available, and Aaron agreed
to take it. As he and I looked at it, he seemed pleased, talking
about furniture and paint color. He slept there for a few weeks,
spending his days as usual, on our couch, or visiting Arthur or
Katherine, when she was free.

According to Arthur, Aaron was mean and ornery.

"Everyone's on Arthur's side uptown," Aaron said.

"Why are there sides?' I asked.

"Because I give him a hard time and insult him."

"His anger provides content," Chris Beels said.

"Intellectual content?" I asked, puzzled.

"Emotional content."

Aaron's comings and goings, his angry denunciations, his
restless dissatisfaction were never far from my thoughts.

Yet there were good moments. Bragging about getting stronger at the gym, I popped out my biceps. Aaron felt the slight bulge they made. "Very butch," he said kindly.

Stasha got a job working with three-year-olds in a summer program at the 14th Street YMHA.

"I think it will be fun," she said. "And it's air-conditioned and it's nearby."

"That's great," I said. "This will be a chance to see how you like being in the classroom." Eight weeks of teaching would keep her busy during the months Jay and I were in Maine.

But as Jay and I prepared to leave a few weeks later, she screamed at me, her face distorted by her distress. "It's easy for you to be happy," she said. "You're going away."

"Is there anything I can do to help?" I asked.

"Just help me end it all."

Her words disturbed and at the same time exasperated me, since I knew she didn't mean them. But I couldn't calm her or elicit any acknowledgment her life was not a wasteland. Her summer job wouldn't work out. She had no money. She had no friends. I was angry at her for giving in to her depression and taking her fears out on me.

We recovered over the course of a weekend. She spent time with Arthur and Lanie and returned home on a more even keel. I let my resentment go.

In Maine Jay was out running the country roads almost daily, preparing for the New York City Marathon in November. We hiked one of our favorite mountains every few days, or found a new one to try. On the phone Stasha complained about her rambunctious three-year-olds at the YMHA summer camp.

Her teenage assistants were also a handful, uncooperative and disrespectful. She phoned to tell me about an awful dispute she had had with them. She had called in the director, who scolded them roundly. But that opened a space for Stasha to talk with them more constructively. She finished by saying, "I hope tomorrow isn't like today. Well, nothing could be as bad as this, so that heartens me." Bravo, Stasha, I thought.

Home again at the end of August, I helped Stasha take her cat to the vet, suspecting that her time had come.

"It's probably a tumor," the vet said. "The only way to know for sure is to run some tests."

Testing and treating eighteen-year-old Felicity made no sense. Stasha and I took turns holding her and said good-bye. Then the vet gave her an injection as she lay in Stasha's arms.

I slung my arm around Stasha's shoulders as we walked home with the empty cat carrier.

"We had her for a long time," I said. "You got her for your sixteenth birthday." Stasha wiped away her tears.

"I'm sorry," Aaron said when we sat down in the living room and told him. "Poor Felicity. Do you want to have a memorial, Stash?"

Stasha shook her head. "We told them to cremate her. No memorial."

Like me, Jay noticed such moments. After Aaron's death, he told of glimpsing the person he had never known one evening as Aaron talked with Stasha about a new computer she meant to buy. Aaron had decided he knew the kind of computer she should get. He had an elaborate theory why this would be good for her. . . . The two of them were sitting on the couch, holding hands, and he kept kind of shaking her hand, and trying every which way to persuade her this computer was going to improve her life and bring her satisfaction and make her a better person. I . . . thought yes. . . . If I saw that outside of everything else I knew, it would have been a brother and sister loving each other and teasing each other.

Aaron wasn't happy in the second-floor studio for long because "something in the air" was giving him a sore throat. When his complaints about the poisoned air continued, Jay and I decided to take the studio as our bedroom but continue to share the living space on the fourth floor with Stasha and Aaron. It was two flights up in the morning and two down again for bed, but we gained a little measure of distance from the difficulties of living with Aaron. With its white walls and high ceiling, its white marble fireplace, and two tall windows overlooking the garden behind the house, the studio was charming and quiet. Jay used the kitchen as a study, placing his desk at the window. On weekends I would find him there, working at his computer or going over student work.

Stasha took the big bedroom we had vacated on the fourth floor, and Aaron the little one. But despite having the rest of us passing in and out, he often slept on the living room couch. He was sure that I was putting something in his food and woke me in the middle of the night to say he had diarrhea as a result. Then he became preoccupied with the idea that he had contracted Lyme disease when he and Katherine had visited Naushon, which was rife with ticks.

Stasha was starting a job as an assistant teacher at First Presbyterian Church Nursery School, where she had subbed in the spring.

Now that she was getting a regular paycheck, she paid a share of household expenses. Sometimes she cooked for us. She stood next to me to help wash and dry dishes and put them away. At last she was chugging through her days in the classroom and her evening studies with some equanimity. She was more sensible and amusing, more expressive and loving than she had been during the long period of her depression. She dealt with Aaron with less anxiety.

"I almost beat Jay at ghost," I told her, referring to a word game he and I played sometimes, which he usually won.

"How boring," Stasha said.

"I think those stupid movies you watch all the time are boring," I said.

"I think those stupid movies you watch are boring," she said.

"I think all the boring things you do are boring," I said. Then we both laughed until we were gasping and then laughed more.

After Aaron and Katherine went together to see the psychiatrist Aaron had seen on his own, he came home and threw himself on the bed in his narrow bedroom. As I passed the door, I saw him lying there, hand on his forehead, thinking. But he didn't confide in me. I had the impression that Katherine had decided it wasn't possible to have a future with him. But her resolve wavered. She loved Aaron, and with her he was at his best. This year she was teaching at a school in Brooklyn and living with her grandmother in a big apartment on the Upper West Side. Aaron couldn't stay with her there, where he would be intruding on a woman in her nineties who was frightened by the crazy person her granddaughter was involved with.

As the fall wore on and Aaron saw Katherine only occasionally, he grew more paranoid and sometimes quite ferociously angry. I asked Stasha to call Katherine to find out what was going on and was upset when I heard her tell Katherine it wasn't safe to live with Aaron. Was that how she felt? I asked her in distress. Clearly, it was—to her Aaron represented a danger. Eventually, Katherine suggested Aaron live at Fountain House, an excellent residential community for the mentally ill. This upset him even more.

Chapter 14

At last Jay and I ended our long dance toward marriage and in December went down to the Municipal Building to be pronounced husband and wife with Weslea as our witness. It felt good, straightforward and uncomplicated. Our marriage became a new feature in my personal geography, perhaps a mountain formed from magma that presses up through the earth's crust from beneath the surface. Or perhaps this new feature was more like mountains formed by the crunching together of two tectonic plates, the plates of my past with Arthur and my love for Jay. In a dream I was flying, using an ability I had developed well, pushing off with my toes and lifting, lifting into the air, coasting over the landscape.

"Congratulations, Ingrid," Aaron said very formally, when I told him Jay and I had married. But he didn't attend the party our friends gave for us, since he rarely socialized with people outside the family. On an occasion when he couldn't avoid a family friend, he amused him by saying, "Just think of me as a very large potted plant." Weslea heard a more typical remark: "Ingrid's a mafioso, they're making a movie about her called the *Godmother*. It's a sequel to *Arsenic and Old Lace*."

I was happy if a visitor who encountered Aaron was able to say something kind; several friends earned my lasting gratitude by remarking on his good looks. Why did that mean so much to me? I think because, although his expression was often angry or depressed, his looks provided the clearest continuity with his past. They were one thing schizophrenia hadn't been able to steal.

Katherine persuaded Aaron to make an appointment with a counselor for people with disabilities at the New York State Department of Labor. As he prepared for his interview, he worked himself into a rant, preventing me and Jay from exchanging a word over our morning coffee. Jay left for his morning class looking miserable. Trying to ignore Aaron, I lay down on the living room carpet to do my exercises.

"It's so embarrassing to watch you prance around," he said.

So I fled to the studio on the second floor.

He returned from his appointment, informing me that the interviewer was a woman who had attended Stuyvesant when he was there. I hurt for him, imagining his discomfort and her awkwardness when she found one of the most brilliant students of her class at Stuyvesant disabled by mental illness.

Increasingly agitated, Aaron woke me from sleep to scold me urgently for feeding him medication that upset his nervous system. The next morning he started in again. He thought the psychiatrist he had seen was supplying Veselka with medication to put in the coffee he bought there. Or perhaps they used rat poison.

"How would they do that?" I asked. "The coffee comes out of that big urn. You're standing right there when they fill your cup."

"Sleight of hand."

"I get coffee there. I feel fine."

"They know I'm vulnerable."

Nothing I said could make a dent in his paranoia. "Things are not as they seem," he told me ominously. When he asked if I would go for genetic testing to prove I was his mother, I agreed readily. He just as quickly lost interest, doubtless thinking that I would manage to falsify the test.

Stasha was disturbed when Aaron woke her one night, standing naked in her doorway, though half-turned away from her, to tell her he was being poisoned. His phone rang as he talked. "It's the phone company," he said, leaving her to wonder why NYNEX would call at three in the morning. Then he dressed and left, saying he was going somewhere safer, which turned out to be Arthur's. But we were all conscious of the level of his fears and agitation, his new delusion that Katherine had other lovers.

It must have been around this time that he wrote to Katherine on several squares of a small note pad, a letter that I think, and hope, he never delivered. Years later I found the bits of paper in the folder with all his Medicare statements and test reports.

Dear Katherine,
. . . I've given up the idea that you'll ever be monogamous or that I can really believe what you say and so I've aban-

doned the idea of marriage and lost all interest in your having children or in being a father. I couldn't adopt and I couldn't get married only to live as a cuckold. I'm sorry that your ob/gyn and you have decided that the decisions that you make about the care of your self have myself as a witness and don't want to deprive you of something that you have to gain from marriage just because I can't deal with the uncertainty of your wishes. . . . . I hope to see you some time w/o the constant frustration of whether or when we'll have sex, and to feel like you don't have to constantly run off all the time seeking solace in zillions of people's arms. Best of wishes.

love, Aaron

A few days later, in one of his attempts to broaden Arthur's horizons, Aaron persuaded him to visit Cuttyhunk, one of the Elizabeth Islands, of which Naushon is the largest. Cuttyhunk, however, is not owned by the Forbes family. Anyone can go there who can take the daily ferry from New Bedford, Massachusetts.

"The ins and outs of why Aaron thought this would be good for me are too convoluted to relate," Arthur said at Aaron's memorial. "But one was his theory that Cuttyhunk is the real jewel of the Elizabeth Islands."

"What was Cuttyhunk like?" I asked Arthur.

"Barren, windy, no trees, very exposed."

I knew the trip must have been trying. But I was sad that Aaron never proposed going anywhere with me. Instead, he treated me with steady animosity, which let up briefly now and then, but never for long enough to go out for so much as lunch, much less a trip together. He treated Arthur similarly, I knew. The difference was that he invited Arthur to go places.

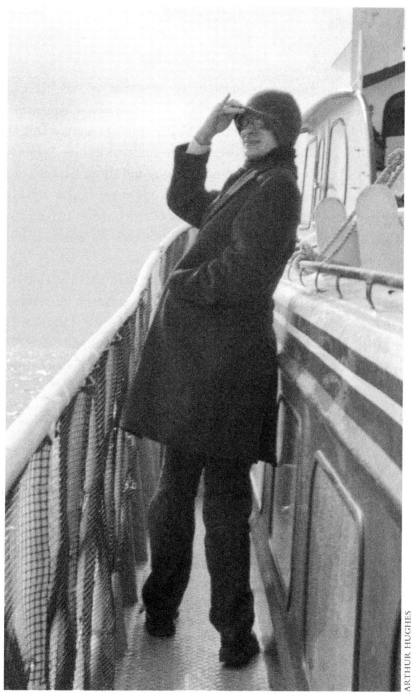

Aaron, Cuttyhunk Ferry, 1999

ARTHUR HUGHES

———

One evening Aaron was seized by the idea that we watched too much television. It wasn't good. We were addicted. He lectured us sternly, then unplugged the TV and started to lug it out to the hall. Vexed, I rose and went to the apartment door to block his way out. He set the television down and stood haranguing me, in a manner threatening enough for Jay to get up and stand behind me, evidently concerned that Aaron would strike out. This occurred to me too, but I couldn't believe Aaron would hurt me.

Jay said later that this was the point when he realized that he couldn't continue with his policy of ignoring Aaron's threatening behavior, the attitude that had served him since Aaron came to live with us. And Aaron's mischief was escalating.

I answered the phone to find a caller asking for Paulo, my downstairs tenant.

"You have the wrong number," I said.

The caller recited a number I knew was Paulo's.

"That's right. Try again," I said, puzzled. But the phone rang again for Paulo. And his number didn't resemble ours, didn't even have the same prefix. I concluded that Aaron had rewired the telephone junction box NYNEX maintained for the building in the cellar.

When a young repairperson came I took him down to the antiquated junction box with its wires sprouting in all directions. He corrected the wiring, politely ignoring what must have been obvious—that someone had deliberately switched the lines. I didn't even bring this up with Aaron, but let it go as one of those inexplicable NYNEX mess-ups.

———

Jay and Stasha had left for work, and I was eating breakfast in our kitchen when Aaron came in and grabbed a bottle of vitamins and another of ibuprofen from a shelf. "There's too much medication around here," he said, dumping them in the trash.

"Aaron. Stop it." But instead he went further. He took my keys from the hook where I always hung them and, lowering the sash, held them out the top half of the kitchen window, as if to let them fall into the courtyard behind the house.

"Don't drop them," I said.

"Why not?"

"Because I need them."

But he let the keys fall. He went off and rummaged in Stasha's closet till he found a bottle of liquid Prozac and emptied it into the sink. This was too far beyond acceptable. Now Stasha would need to replace her medication. I would have to retrieve my keys before I left for BMCC. But first I had to deal with Aaron. Putting my feelings on hold, I went into coping mode.

"I could call the police," I said matter-of-factly.

"I'll call the police on you."

"You can't do that."

"I can do anything short of assault you."

"No, you can't."

"Go ahead. Call them."

"It's a big step. I won't do it till I think it over."

Then I ran down the stairs and had to wake young Paulo by leaning on his buzzer. He raised his eyebrows, but spared me from explaining how my keys could have fallen out the window. I let myself out his back door and picked them up.

Before I left the house to teach, I called Arthur. He too felt Aaron's behavior was no longer tolerable.

"Call the police," he said.

"What hospital should I send him to?"

"Saint Vincent's."

He and I both understood that calling 911 would mean a hospital evaluation for Aaron. It was the one avenue we hadn't been able to pursue. Perhaps Aaron's behavior now would qualify him for hospitalization. At this point Arthur and I were both ready for it, though I grumbled to myself, perhaps unfairly, that Arthur wanted me to be the heavy.

As I returned from my class, Stasha was coming in from her nursery school. I told her what had happened. Aaron listened, standing in the living room doorway as he ran a bath.

"I'm going to call the police," I said, addressing them both.

"Please do. I'll dial for you." Aaron moved toward the phone, his long arm reaching for it, but as a gesture only, before he went off to bathe. Stasha went to her room.

Alone, I picked up the phone. The long history of Aaron's illness lay behind my resolution to call 911. "My son is psychotic and we need an ambulance to take him to the hospital," I said.

"Is he raving? Does he have a weapon? Is he violent?"

"No. No. No."

"Keep him calm, ma'am."

As Aaron was splashing in the tub, Stasha reappeared.

"I called the police."

"Aren't you going to tell Aaron?"

"OK, tell him."

Stasha went to the bathroom door. "Aaron. Mom called the police."

"What?"

"Mom called the police."

Aaron got out of the tub and stood in the living room doorway, wrapped in a towel, wet and naked, holding his clothes. I

202

hadn't considered how vulnerable he must feel. But then I wasn't considering my own feelings either, but keeping to my plan, one step at a time.

"You called the police?"

"Yes."

He went to his room to dress. The buzzer sounded. In the hall I intercepted two strapping, blue-uniformed policemen mounting the stairs. There was no way I was going to let them near Aaron. Seeing them would make him far more upset. They waited in the hall, quite willing to leave dealing with a psychotic young man to the EMTs, who soon arrived. I took them into Aaron's room, where he was dressed and sitting on the futon. One started questioning him as Stasha and I stood near the bedroom door listening. When asked why he had thrown away Stasha's medication, Aaron said, "She takes too many supplements."

"You have a point there," the man said.

I was too upset to smile. At least the medic was trained to deal with the situation, I thought gratefully.

After twenty minutes the EMT needed to move Aaron along.

"If you won't come with us on your own, we'll have to take you forcibly," he said. Aaron picked up his pack and let them escort him away.

"Go with him," I told Stasha. She followed them down to the street.

Hanging out the front window, I watched as they walked him to the ambulance. He climbed in, turning Stasha away. "He was trembling," she said when she was back.

Now I was free to sit quietly for a while. But I was too upset. I wanted to be near Aaron. I had called an ambulance not as a way to distance him, but in the hope that a hospital psychiatrist might lead us in a new direction. So a little later we walked across town to Saint Vincent's. Aaron was sitting on the edge of a bed in the hall wearing a hospital gown, so pale his lips were blue. A nurse had a blood pressure cuff around his biceps.

"Here's the woman who's responsible for me being here," he said.

"Mom?" the nurse asked.

I nodded. "I brought you a toothbrush," I said, handing it over with a tube of paste.

"OK. You can leave now," he said, dismissing me.

Stasha headed uptown and I walked home alone, reviewing the events of the day, anxious but still holding my feelings in check. I had done what I thought needed to be done, though it was awful to think of Aaron being taken away, so pale and scared. Still, if Saint Vincent's would keep him, that might help. But we weren't there yet.

Through the evening my sense of crisis continued as I got one call after another. The psychiatrist Aaron had seen wanted me to know she had heard from him. She had encouraged the hospital psychiatrist to keep him, saying he had threatened me. That was the point that mattered, even though I didn't feel the television episode constituted a threat. Later Arthur let me know Aaron had been released and was on his way to Arthur's.

I wasn't surprised that Aaron could pass psychiatric muster—I had known calling 911 was a long shot. But I was disappointed.

A few hours later Aaron called. "There's something bad in the air here. I'm coming downtown. I want you to know I'll never forgive you."

If he was returning, I needed to see him. So I climbed the stairs in my bathrobe and dozed off on the couch until I heard the bolt on the door turning. Aaron stretched out on the opposite couch.

"What happened?" I asked, sitting up.

"The psychiatrist asked why I was there. I said I was having a dispute with my mother about the exact line I had to cross before EMS would take me away. Which I lost."

Small wonder the psychiatrist had released him after hearing that sentence. Quite apart from its structure, it revealed Aaron's clear understanding of the incident that had led me to call 911. As Arthur and I had, he saw there was a line he had crossed.

Even while I was exhausted by worrying and phone calls interrupting my sleep, I laughed at Aaron's report. Stasha laughed too when she appeared in her coat to go to teach her four-year-olds. As Aaron rolled over to sleep, he said, "Don't ever do that again, Ingrid."

"I won't, if you don't throw my keys out the window."

We spoke with candor and intimacy, the characteristics of our relationship from Aaron's childhood.

Shoving a cushion under my head, I slept as well.

As it became increasingly difficult to function with Aaron in the house, my therapist said she thought I shouldn't let him live with us. I found it hard to bring this up with Chris Beels when Arthur and I next saw him. But I did. And I brought it up with Aaron. I gave him no deadline, but said I'd like him to find another place to live.

Katherine came over a few days after my attempt to have Aaron hospitalized. She was downtown waiting for visiting hours at NYU Medical Center, where her grandmother was hospitalized.

"Aaron tells me he's broken up with you," I said, though her presence contradicted his report. She laughed. Then Aaron went uptown and spent the night with her, since her grandmother wasn't home. He left on a bus tour of the Midwest a few evenings later, in a state of rage, after sputtering and flaring all day long. From the bus he called me.

"I'll never forgive you. You're ignoble," he said, still bitter over being taken to the hospital against his will.

I understand now how frightened he was to be in the custody, even briefly, of the medical system he so often reviled. Then, his anger seemed no different from his usual hostility. So the sorrow I felt as he set off on his travels around the country was mixed with relief to have quiet in the house after the weeks of his agitation.

Arthur got messages from Toledo, Ohio, and South Bend, Indiana, as the bus carried Aaron across the country. At one point he called his old friend Philip in Colorado, though he hadn't seen him for years. Ten days after his departure, I came home to find him soaking in the bathtub. As always, I was glad he was home.

As I thought about how distressed Aaron was, it crossed my mind that suicide was a possibility. I reassured myself by going back to my conversation with Dr. White years before, when I told him Aaron found the idea of suicide shocking. White had thought that was a good indication. That had been seven years ago, but I clung to the memory.

It's easy now to arrange this story to show how Aaron's illness developed, and easy, at many points, to wish I had acted differently. Perhaps I could have prevented Aaron's death if . . . And if . . . And if. These wishes give an illusion of control. But they deny reality. There were reasons I acted as I did. Good or bad, they determined my choices. There were reasons for his choice. Stark and absolute as it is, I have to live with what happened.

Chapter 15

I said good-bye to the duty officer at the Paris embassy, hung up the phone, and sat in silence with Stasha. When we pulled ourselves together enough to go upstairs, Stasha called Arthur. Soon he and Lanie were with us.

"If Stasha keeps on crying, I'm going to go crazy," I muttered to Lanie as Arthur and Stasha embraced and cried. I could hardly bear their pain.

The four of us sat in the living room, stunned and quiet: Lanie with her Jewish Afro, nicely dressed as always in slacks and a sweater; Arthur, whose hair and thick eyebrows were white now; Stasha, substantial and sad. My anxiety lay on me, a painful mantle, searing my spine, tightening my shoulders.

I couldn't tell Jay; he had taken my nephew and niece, who were visiting for spring break, to the Museum of Natural History. Now and then it would occur to Arthur or Lanie or me that we had to tell someone what had happened; we would go to the phone. My shock and disorientation were so great that

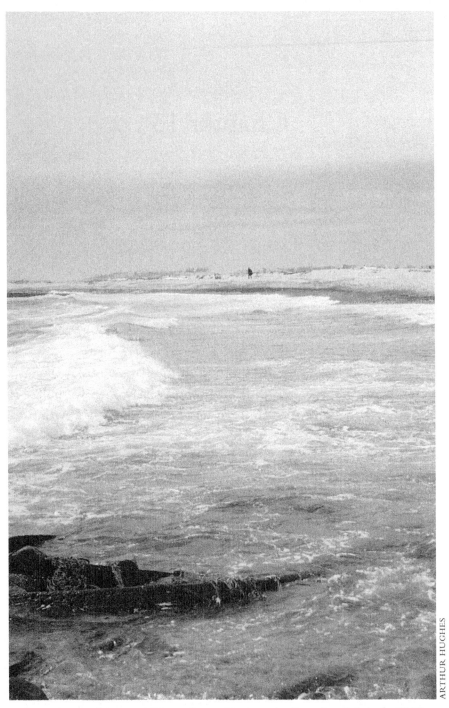

Last photo of Aaron (distant figure in center), Cuttyhunk beach, 1999

when I called my brother David, it was not because I realized I had to tell him Aaron had died, but to explain that his kids would be returning home earlier than planned. Then I thought to call my father, and he took over calling family.

Late in the afternoon Jay returned with Ben and Stephanie to find us still sitting. He stared at me as I explained what had happened.

"I never thought how he must be feeling," he said, acknowledging how hard the last months had been for him.

Arthur, who had avoided meeting Jay all these years, rose to introduce himself. They shook hands, Jay looking bewildered. I was grateful for Arthur's gesture that said he was ready to accept Jay's role in the family.

Katherine was away with her mother on a cycling trip for the week of spring break. After some debate with myself, I told her father. That evening she called, crying so hard I could hardly understand her. I told her what we had learned from the duty officer at the Embassy.

"I waited so long for him," she said as she sobbed. "I waited for so many years."

"I know," I said. "I know."

"Do you think we'll get a letter?" she asked.

"You might. I don't think we will." I was sure Aaron wouldn't have felt a need to explain to us.

While Katherine wanted a letter, what I wanted was to feel Aaron had loved me. A dream gave me that, a dream that Aaron died, then came alive again to say, "I want you to know that I love you." He smiled, and then he died again. His words seemed real and true: of course, he loved me.

For days people moved in and out of our apartment, stopping for a short visit or a long one, sitting singly or in groups. The years of being alone with Aaron's illness, of people's clumsy remarks that came of not understanding, were over now. Friends brought food; they asked if there was anything they could do. Weslea went with me to Saint Mark's Church to arrange for the memorial. Arthur found an undertaker in New York who could work with a French undertaker to arrange for the return of Aaron's body. He had a friend in Paris take flowers to the Buttes-Chaumont and leave them on the bridge near the tree Aaron had chosen to hang himself from. This near-stranger talked with a park worker who had seen Aaron's body. "Such a shame. Such a handsome man," the park worker said.

Sometimes I cried. Often I felt battered, as if I had been tossed into the air and whacked around. Descending the stairs or the front stoop, I feared tumbling down. A sense of anger and horror rose in me whenever I thought of Stasha's footsteps on the stairs, her cries for me, her message that Aaron was dead. It was a long time before I realized that those feelings were inevitable and had nothing to do with Stasha.

But Aaron was free now—free of the poisons and toxic fumes, the lies and people in league against him. Shattering as his death was, it freed me too. We had lost him years earlier, when he lost his mind, an expression I had come to regard as a rather exact description of his illness. The years of disorder and confusion were over, and I could remember him as himself.

At the same time I was deeply grateful for his year and a half at home with us. How terrible it would have been if he had ended his life in Boston, as Katherine now told us he had tried to do. How glad I was for his brilliant, berserk presence at home in his last year and a half. Despite his belligerence and his mischief, despite the beating I took, his presence provided a restoration of our intimacy. At every step, it was better to have had Aaron in our lives. It would have been a far greater loss not to have had him, not to have loved him.

Stasha too felt relieved, I saw, as the days passed. Arthur was inconsolable. Katherine was in terrible pain, angry at herself, and at us, though she never quite said as much. Her longing for Aaron was powerful and lasting. I had a sense that she had an alternative to his death worked out in her head, in which she found a way to live with him and take care of him. I believed that if he had lived with her, he would have turned against her. The delusion that she had other lovers would have been followed by others, making him hostile and belligerent. But she had loved him and known him well. I couldn't argue with her feelings

On the morning of the memorial, we set up the sanctuary of Saint Mark's Church. We spread a table with a sheet Aaron had tie-dyed in pink suns during his time with the Nicaragua Construction Brigade. Arthur's photographs of Aaron and the family went on the table. Arthur's sister set out bunches of pale green and mauve flowers.

As I walked the two blocks from 311 later in the day, I met first one friend and then another on the street, and then in the church, and everyone hugged me. It felt so good, comfort I had longed for since he got sick.

Arthur's family had come from Boston and California, my siblings and nieces and nephews from Washington and Pennsylvania; my New York cousins were present, Aaron's friend Philip came from Colorado; Katherine's parents and siblings and their families were present, and Aaron's friends from high school. My father stood talking to people, his head the highest as we got ready to begin. Speaking about Aaron to this audience, I was comforted by knowing I didn't have to explain how remarkable he had been. They knew. I insisted that we respect Aaron's decision to take his life.

I understood his choice not as a way to accuse us, but to leave his pain behind. Yet it was hard to sleep. I tried different drugstore remedies and prescriptions from Chris Beels. But I would find myself going over the last weeks in my head, wanting to remember the details of his last days. If I did succeed in falling asleep, I would wake from nightmares in a terror that thrummed through my body, then gradually died back to lie in my gut.

It took ten days for the French undertaker to get Aaron's body in its cardboard case on a plane. At the funeral parlor on Bleecker Street, he lay in a dark coffin in the clothes he had died in, washed and clean. After dreading the sight of his body, I found I didn't want to leave him. His face was not quite right around the mouth, but definitely him, dead and final, and still handsome, his hair a little longer than it had been when he left New York, his arms at his sides as when he hung from the tree. His belt was worn and his waist narrow; he hadn't eaten much the last days. He looked long in the casket.

He wanted this, I told myself, as I cried. He wanted us to see his body shockingly empty of him, empty of his madness, of his wit, of his anguish. Standing at his head, I ran my fingers through his hair. Stasha tucked her scarf in by his hand. I was glad he seemed whole, though I knew that this was because the marks of the rope had been carefully covered by his turtleneck.

Arthur and I watched them screw the coffin shut. In the limousine we rode in silence after the hearse to the damp spring graveyard where the trees were just beginning to leaf. They lowered the coffin into the ground. I read lines from Whitman: "Did we think victory great? So it is—but now it seems to me, when it cannot be helped, that defeat is great, and that death and dismay are great." Arthur and Lanie and Jay all had something to read. Katherine and Stasha sang "'Tis a gift to be free." We each took the spade and shoveled dirt from the sandy heap into the deep cut in the ground. Arthur sobbed quietly as he threw in one spadeful after another, heaving the dirt onto the coffin as if the labor relieved him.

At BMCC, when other teachers offered condolences, I tried to tell them how wonderful Aaron had been, longing for them to know his intelligence and kindness, to be again the mother of a brilliant, lovely young man. In the classroom I focused on my students, a helpful distraction from my grief. As time passed and I was able to think of other things, the thought of Aaron would come to me as I approached our front door, when I sat on the couch where he lay so often, or later at the moment I got into bed.

Aaron's bedroom on the fourth floor was empty. This was the room we had set aside for him, the room where he had often slept, despite objecting that it wasn't his, where he and Katherine had spent his last night at home. He had yanked himself violently out of our world. As Jay helped me move my desk in, I felt the air still shuddering with the shock waves of his death.

I kept his backpack and wool overcoat in the closet—they had come back to us in the temporary coffin the French undertaker had used to ship him home. The pack held his canceled passport, a change of underwear and socks, his toothbrush and paste, the night guard the dentist had made to prevent him from grinding his teeth in his sleep, and most heartbreakingly, a jar of a fiber supplement for that homeliest of vexations, constipation.

Aaron was gone, and I had taken his space. But now that he had no space he was everywhere—on the mountains when we hiked in Maine; in Veselka when I had coffee there; at Saint Mark's when I walked along 10th Street.

What we had of Aaron now were many photos, a few items of clothing, some of his handiwork, a pair of bookends of cherry that he had made during his carpentry days, artwork and craft projects from school, the boxes of his schoolwork in the cellar. I especially liked to have the small, neatly worked sundial he had made in metal shop at Stuyvesant, the three-inch koala bear he was fond of in early childhood. But beyond those leavings, he existed now in our memories, in what we knew of him, along with many questions we would never answer.

In Maine I transcribed the tapes of Aaron's memorial for the book Arthur and I were making for family and friends. I kept my journal so diligently and prosaically that my dreams made fun of me, presenting me with a woman who died and left a literary legacy of a very complete record of the weather in all the places where she had lived. Hiking our favorite mountain trails, it was hard to avoid thinking how easy it would be for someone to throw himself to a rocky death.

It came to me gradually that Aaron had planned his death in advance. The more I thought, the more I understood that he had been considering killing himself for some time. In retrospect, the view that makes fools of us all, the signs I had missed were all too plain. But even Chris Beels, even my therapist, even Stasha's therapist, hadn't recognized them. We had seen Aaron's increasingly troublesome behavior as a problem for us rather than an expression of his despair.

Months earlier I had been sitting in the living room when Aaron constructed one of his passive sentences, facing away from me: "It makes you think there's no sense going on."

"If you did anything it would be terrible for me and Arthur

and Stasha." I didn't understand the need to take this announce-
ment seriously. I don't think I even mentioned it to Chris Beels.

Later Aaron said he was going to West Virginia.

"Why West Virginia?"

"It's easy to get a gun there."

"You'd better not hurt anyone, Aaron."

"I'm not going to hurt anyone," he said quietly. When he
came home from West Virginia, I checked his backpack while
he was out. No gun. I reported what he had said to Chris Beels,
who frowned in distress but evidently didn't catch on either.

Aaron stood in the living room doorway and said, "I want to
do something significant." Something to expand his lot in life
beyond the "incredibly miniscule," he meant, something people
would notice. He grew more agitated. Stasha was so uneasy after
my effort to have him hospitalized that she had a bolt installed
on her bedroom door. Wanting to talk to her after she was asleep,
he tried to break it. She threatened to call the police again. He
grabbed his overcoat and pack and ran off. From bed I heard
footsteps on the stairs, then a whack on the door to Jay's and my
room, more downward pounding and a slam of the door out of
the house. I didn't know what was going on till Stasha explained
in the morning.

Aaron's thump on the door stayed with me, his inarticulate
and angry good-bye. Next day he called from Boston. On his
return he booked a ticket to Paris. Knowing he was leaving
soon, I spent more time with him. He was calmer and we could
talk more.

"What's going on with Katherine?" I asked him.

"She wants me to deal"—he groped for words—"with this
disability thing."

"So?"

"So I did send off an application to one of the places I got from the Department of Labor."

A week or two after his death, this application came back to us, unopened, because it had been misaddressed, one of the possibilities that were no longer possible.

"You seem so sincere, Ingrid," Aaron said. "Now's the time for you to confess."

"Confess what?"

"Are you really my mother?"

"I'm your mother."

I was sitting near his feet as he lay on the couch. "Your left nostril is bigger than your right," I said. "Like Arthur's."

"I don't like to talk about that." He rejected this evidence that Arthur was his father.

As he prepared to leave, Aaron made an appointment with the psychiatrist he had seen. But when he got to her office, she wasn't there. Later she called, saying he should have waited, she was just a bit behind schedule. By then it was too late. Aaron was booked to leave New York for Paris the next day.

We were standing in the door to his room when he said, "I'm depressed and discouraged, demobilized, demilitarized, and zoned out." He was looking past me, toward the window. I appreciated his string of words without understanding. He repeated them: "Depressed and dejected and impotent, demobilized, demilitarized, and zoned out." He meant he was so depressed he was going to zone out entirely. He had said years earlier that he was powerless; he had no choices. Taking his own life seemed to him the only power left. Without the gun he had sought, he was also demilitarized. And demobilized by his decision to take himself out of the fray, to abandon motion, emotion, life.

I got up early on Aaron's last morning at home so I could say good-bye. Through the crack of his half-open door, I could see him holding Katherine in his arms, stroking her shoulder. I turned away silently. She slipped out to go to work while I was in the kitchen. A few minutes later Aaron was putting on his coat.

"Let me go down with you." I wanted to walk him to the subway.

"That would be unfortunate." He was in a fury, out the door already. I stood on the landing as he ran down the stairs. "See you in the next life," he spat at me.

As I straightened up the apartment to prepare for my niece and nephew, I continued to think of Aaron. I had said I would deposit some money in his checking account. "You'd better do that," he told me. So maybe he wasn't completely sure he would take his own life, even then. I made the deposit, wondering if he would be back soon, like the last times he went away.

Next day he landed in Paris, as Stasha and I took her cousins to the Statue of Liberty. We were waiting in line to get in when he bought the rope. The receipt they found in his shirt said five o'clock in the afternoon. He must have gone to the Buttes-Chaumont to choose a tree and find a secluded place to make the noose and the knot. He would have researched how before he left New York. Probably he walked around, too agitated to sit, as he waited for dark and for solitude.

Aaron must have set his little felt pack at the foot of the tree, climbed the trunk in the dark, and attached his rope to a strong limb. He had told Katherine he was terrified. His heart must have been pounding, his hands shaking and sweaty. He put the noose over his head. Did he hesitate? Did he have to force himself to keep on with his plan? He had to adjust the rope around his neck before he dropped from the branch. Then it caught his weight. His neck snapped.

He didn't know that his body in his dark clothes jerked and swung over the water, at first in wild arcs created by his jump, then in smaller and smaller ones, until it became still and his long arms hung at his sides, his capable, strong hands no longer shaking.

Afterword

Seven years after Aaron's death, we celebrated Stasha's marriage to Sotiris Melissis, a Greek composer she had met while teaching at a Greek church school. She and I waited together for Arthur and Sotiris to bring his parents and sister and brother-in-law from the airport. How should I greet Sotiris's parents, these strangers who were so closely connected to me? Do you embrace someone you've never met? Do you shake hands? When Sotiris's mother, Eugenia, stepped in the door and kissed me on both cheeks, I felt like crying, I was so happy—for Stasha, for myself, and for this mother who like me was here to witness her child marry at forty.

Eugenia began to talk to me in Greek, confident that I would understand her. She insisted that Sotiris's sister open their luggage and bring out their gifts, though it was late and I thought she must be exhausted from the long flight and the time change. But she dug into a suitcase and produced two intricately worked white coverlets she had crocheted—one for me and Jay, one for

Arthur and Lanie. A bigger, more elaborate one made by Sotiris's grandmother had been set aside long ago for him and his
bride. I found these gifts entirely satisfying as gestures of respect
and connection.

Stasha and Sotiris lived now in the renovated garden apartment of 311. We held the family dinner in their garden. As dark
fell and we chatted with our relatives, fireflies flickered overhead, as if casting a benediction on Stasha and Sotiris.

At their wedding party, Stasha was svelte and elegant in an
ivory sheath, her hair twisted up behind her head, showing off
her narrow head and lovely face. Katherine attended with her
husband, Joe. The traditional Greek band played the line dances
Stasha and I had been learning from a friend of Sotiris's. Late in
the evening Stasha danced her solo, *kalamatianos,* and later still
Sotiris danced his. Even in my happiness, I was aware of Aaron's
absence and had to fight tears whenever I was moved.

Since Aaron's death, Arthur's elaborately imagined landscapes
invariably included a small Aaron figure and a fantastic, threatening element as well: an animal like a dinosaur looming, an
impossibly huge sea creature emerging from the water, a rock-
scape of huge boulders dwarfing a tiny Aaron. Arthur's work
had been exhibited in Washington, DC, in California, and most
recently at a synagogue in Washington Heights. But I had not
been able to write about Aaron. My one effort, during a summer in Maine, had ended before it began, when I took out my
notes on phone talks with Aaron and read his pleas that I stop
what was happening to him. A quick glance told me I couldn't
deal with it. I put the folder away and went off to the public
library to sink into the alternate universe of a novel. After that
I didn't try to write about him.

———

I was in the delivery room when Stasha brought Iliana into the world, a tiny, lusty new person. That semester I reduced my teaching load so I could help Stasha. After breakfast I would descend from the fourth floor to sit with her as she held Iliana to her breast to nurse, or I would cradle Iliana's warm body in my arms, freeing Stasha to shower or catch up on her sleep. Then I would gaze at Iliana's thatch of dark hair, her plump cheeks, her little shell ears and the shape of her head, as I had gazed at Stasha and then Aaron. Stasha and I noted how fat her legs were getting, how round her belly, how strongly she belted out her song, the eternal cry of babies to the world: I'm here, I'm here, I'm here. "We could call her Lungs," Stasha said. Sotiris measured her bellow at seventy-five decibels. Her smiles would flit over her face when I met her and Stasha on the street, Iliana in a canvas marsupial against Stasha's belly. As Stasha recovered from the delivery, it was clear that she too was thriving. Despite a high level of maternal anxiety, she was energetic and confident.

That season items I had misplaced and forgotten or thought lost forever began to show up, giving me a sense of regaining parts of myself. Iliana was three months old, a thriving new life, when I found the courage to write about Aaron, nine years after his death. I reread Amos Oz's story of his life and his mother's suicide, *A Tale of Love and Darkness*, one of my inspirations for this book. In Maine that summer, I was able to sketch out this story very briefly from beginning to end.

In order to write, I studied Aaron's life and my own, gathering materials and sifting them, using my memory to weave them into a narrative. Often I felt I had upended the past into the present, where it lay in the piles of my notebooks and Aar-

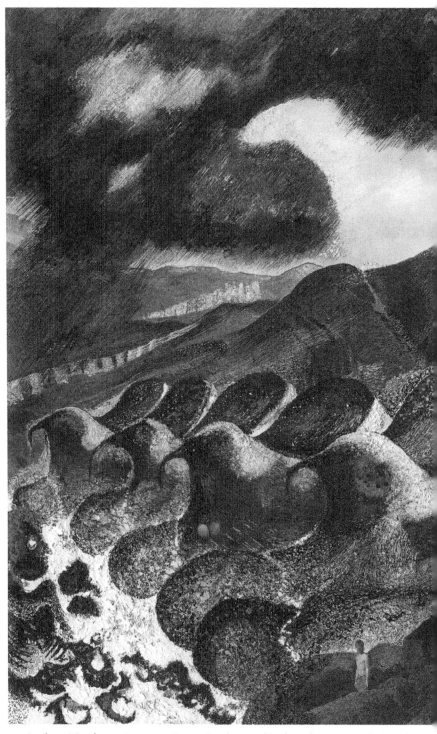

Arthur Hughes, *Aaron at Sespe Creek*, acrylic, brush, pen-and-Epson ink on inkjet paper

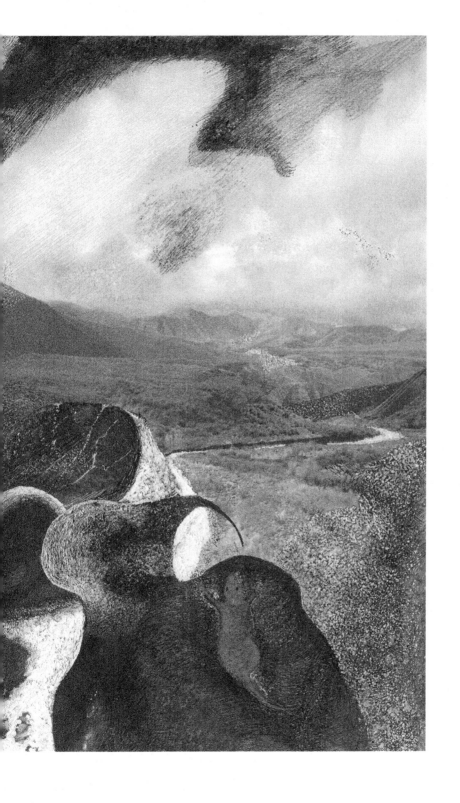

on's on my table. Dreams from the years of Aaron's illness I was dreaming again: Aaron was a child in a stroller, Aaron was an adult but his deranged self. Or I was parting from Arthur with much ambivalence and many postmortem reconsiderations. At times I couldn't bear to be alone at home with my past and went to the library to read or off to a movie.

Aaron's high school journals, which I found a year or two into my project, gave me his voice, and renewed my sense of him and his sensible, matter-of-fact intelligence and kindness. Working with them restored his long ago gift to me, the space for Ingridity, which has grown larger as I've been writing his story. At the same time, reviewing Aaron's life dug up a lot of grief. No matter how many times I resolved to avoid the falseness of imagining a happier, better past, I couldn't help seeing where I could have done better. Fearing that readers would judge me as I was judging myself, I wondered if I could skip over those errors in judgment. But I couldn't. They are part of the story.

My sorrow at the way we lost Aaron remains part of me, along with a deep appreciation of the person he was and an abiding gratitude for the time when he was part of our lives.

Resources

The National Alliance on Mental Illness (NAMI), offers peer-led support groups, community programs, state conferences and a national convention every year. Look for an affiliate near you at https://www.nami.org/Find-Your-Local-NAMI
The American Foundation for Suicide Prevention. afsp.org. AFSP works to raise awareness, offer support, fund research and call for a national response to the problem of suicide.

Many books about understanding mental illness and many memoirs are available at your bookstore and library. I have listed only a few.

Amador, Xavior. *I Am Not Sick I Don't Need Help! How to Help Someone with Mental Illness to Accept Treatment.* Vida Press, 2010. A program to talk a family member or friend into trying treatment without antagonizing her or him.
Chase, Ronald. *Schizophrenia: A Brother Finds Answers in Biolog-*

ical Science. Baltimore, MD: Johns Hopkins University Press, 2013. Chapters on the life of Chase's older brother alternate with chapters on the science of schizophrenia as of 2013.

Cockburn, Patrick, and Henry Cockburn. *Henry's Demons: Living with Schizophrenia, a Father and Son's Story.* New York: Scribner, 2011. The story of Henry's illness with chapters by his father and Henry himself.

Ginsberg, Allen. *Kaddish and Other Poems, 1958–1960.* San Francisco: City Lights Books,1960. A long poem in memory of Ginsberg's mother, who suffered from schizophrenia.

Greenberg, Michael. *Hurry Down Sunshine.* New York: Other Press, 2008. Greenberg describes his teenage daughter's acute onset of mania.

Hoss, Phoebe. *All Eyes: A Mother's Struggle to Save Her Schizophrenic Son.* Durham, NC: Carolina Wren Press, 2011. The story of a boy who had symptoms of schizophrenia from childhood and ended by taking his own life.

Kaye, Randye. *Ben Behind His Voices: One Family's Journey from the Chaos of Schizophrenia to Hope.* Lanham, MD: Rowman & Littlefield, 2011. A mother's story of her son's illness.

Lewis, Mindy. *Life Inside: A Memoir.* New York: Washington Square Press, 2002. Lewis was committed to a mental hospital in her teens, despite her lack of major mental illness. This is the story of her three years in hospital.

Mueser, Kim T., and Susan Gengerich. *The Complete Family Guide to Schizophrenia: Helping Your Loved One Get the Most Out of Life.* New York: Guilford Press, 2006. A guide for families.

Neugeboren, Jay. *Imagining Robert: My Brother, Madness, and Survival: A Memoir.* New York: William Morrow, 1997. Neugeboren writes about his own life and that of his schizophrenic brother.

————. *Transforming Madness: New Lives for People Living with Mental Illness.* New York: William Morrow, 1999.

North, Carol. *Welcome Silence: My Triumph Over Schizophrenia.* New York: Simon & Schuster,1987. North describes living with schizophrenia from childhood and a rare type of cure.

Oz, Amos. *A Tale of Love and Darkness.* San Diego: Harcourt-Books.com, 2004. The Israeli writer tells the story of his life and of his mother's depression and suicide.

Saks, Elyn R. *The Center Cannot Hold: My Journey Through Madness.* New York: Hyperion, 2008. A memoir by a professor of law who lives with schizophrenia.

Schiller, Lori, with Amanda Bennett. *The Quiet Room: A Journey Out of the Torment of Madness.* New York: Warner Books, 1994. Schiller tells of living with schizophrenia, many hospitalizations, and finally a doctor who helped her recover.

Styron, William. *Darkness Visible: A Memoir of Madness,* New York: Random House, 1990. Styron describes his major depression and how he recovered.

Torrey, E. Fuller. *Surviving Schizophrenia: A Family Manual.* 6th edition. New York: Harper Perennial, 2013. A comprehensive resource discussing many aspects of schizophrenia and the problems of those who live with it and their families.

Vonnegut, Mark. *The Eden Express: A Memoir of Insanity.* New York: Praeger, 1975.

————. *Just Like Someone Without Mental Illness Only More So.* New York: Bantam Books, 2010. *The Eden Express* is a sixties story of several breakdowns, remarkable for its description of what goes on in the head of a person who is psychotic. *Just Like Someone Without Mental Illness* was written later in life takes a longer view.

Acknowledgments

My thanks go to Mindy Lewis, who read an embryonic version of this story and suggested I develop it into a book, then read drafts of many chapters and decorated them all with extensive and supportive marginal comments. I also had the benefit of thoughtful responses from C. Christian Beels, Stephanie Ellis, Wendy Fairey, Joyce Gallagher, Carol Gaskin, Nancy Hoch, Linda Mockler, Marcia Newfield, Sue Ribner, Wendy Scribner, Jeff Traite, and Christine Wade.

Meredith Sue Willis has been unfailing source of friendship and writerly encouragement over many years, and in addition read several drafts of this book and provided important feedback.

Arthur Hughes answered endless questions about our life with Aaron and Stasha and commented helpfully on an early draft. His photos and paintings of Aaron are an essential part of Aaron's story. For more of them go to arthurhughes.net.

Philip Lidov, Katherine Sorel, Susanna Siegel, and Stasha

228

Hughes provided me with useful reminiscenses of Aaron, and answered my questions as well as they could. Their memories helped me understand Aaron. His Swarthmore professors, Amy Bug, now Amy Graves, and John Bocce, have kindly allowed me to quote from their letters.

Most central is Jay Klokker, whose presence, patience, and careful reading have been essential to my writing.

CPSIA information can be obtained
at www.ICGtesting.com
Printed in the USA
BVOW09s0053051217
501912BV00016B/82/P

9 780990 376736